statnote:
dot phrases to expedite your medical documentation

primary care phrase library

1000+ boilerplate templates

FIRST EDITION

GERARDO GUERRA BONILLA, MD
Copyright © 2019 by Gerardo Guerra Bonilla, MD

All rights reserved.

ISBN: 9781081360184

All rights reserved. This book is protected by copyright. No part of this book may be reproduced in any form by any means, including as photocopies or scanned-in or other electronic copies, or utilized by any information storage and retrieval system without written permission from the copyright owner, except for brief quotations embodied in critical articles
and reviews. To request permission, please contact StatNote at 2233 Watt Ave, Suite 282, PMB 14097, Sacramento, CA 95825, via email at support@statnote.com, or via our website at statnote.com.

This work is provided "as is," and the publisher disclaims any and all warranties, express or implied, including any warranties as to accuracy, comprehensiveness or currency of the content of this work. This work is no substitute for individual patient assessment based upon healthcare professionals' examination of each patient and consideration of, among other things, age, weight, gender, current or prior medical conditions, medication history, laboratory data and other factors unique to the patient. The publisher does not provide medical advice or guidance, and this work is merely a reference tool. Healthcare professionals, and not the publisher, are solely responsible for the use of this work, including all medical judgments and for any resulting diagnoses and treatments.

Given continuous, rapid advances in medical science and health information, independent professional verification of medical diagnoses, indications, appropriate pharmaceutical selections and dosages, and treatment options should be made, and healthcare professionals should consult a variety of sources. When prescribing medication, healthcare professionals are advised to consult the product information sheet (the manufacturer's package insert) accompanying each drug to verify, among other things, conditions of use, warnings and side effects and identify any changes in dosage schedule or contraindications, particularly if the medication to be administered is new, infrequently used or has a narrow therapeutic range. All templates (also known as autotext, dot phrases, smart phrases), procedure reports or other text found in this book are intended as examples only. Documentation in the medical record should always reflect precisely the specific interaction with an individual patient. Failure to carefully review and update any content used from these templates can endanger patients and increase liability risk. To the maximum extent permitted under applicable law, no responsibility is assumed by the publisher for any injury and/or damage to persons or property, as a matter of product liability, negligence law or otherwise, or from any reference to or use by any person of this work.

DEDICATION

To my parents Gerardo and Blanca. To my best friend and the love of my life Lauren. To my lovely children Marco, Emilia and Mateo.

CONTENTS

	Acknowledgments	v
	Foreword	vi
	Preface	vii
	Introduction	viii
1	General Medicine	1
	1.1 Billing Codes	11
	1.2 Health Maintenance/Physicals	16
	1.3 Physical Exam	29
2	Cardiology	32
3	Dermatology	38
4	Endocrinology	69
5	ENT and Ophthalmology	73
6	Gastroenterology	87
7	Hematology/Oncology	92
8	Infectious Diseases	94
9	Neurology	102
10	OB/GYN	118

statnote dot phrases - primary care phrase library

11	Musculoskeletal (ortho/sports/podiatry)	136
12	Pediatrics	184
13	Psychology	214
14	Pulmonology	226
15	Renal/Urology	230
16	Surgery	239
	16.1 Billing Codes	254
17	Urgent Care	264
18	Inpatient/SNF	274
	18.1 Billing Codes	283
19	Messages: Lab, Imaging, Path Results	291
20	Miscellaneous	305
	Subject Index	321
	About the Author	330

ACKNOWLEDGMENTS

Special thanks to all my career mentors for their profound influence in my personal and professional life. I will always be grateful for your support and kindness.

I also appreciate the editing support of Mark McFarlane.

FOREWORD

In 2016, Gerardo was a resident at the Dignity Northridge Family Medicine Residency where I had the good fortune of being his program director. Gerardo always impressed me because he pushed boundaries to find ways for physicians to do their work in a more efficient and timely manner.

All residents were required to complete a scholarly project. Many chose diabetes or hypertension, but Gerardo decided to do his assignment on the patient's perception of the physician utilizing an off-site scribe to type notes in real time through technology used during the office visit. He was diligent when there were barriers to his project, revised his goals as needed and persevered. His findings revealed that most patients understood the benefit to have an off-site virtual scribe help with computer documentation.

Gerardo graduated and today is a practicing family medicine physician. This past year our group followed his lead and started using remote scribes for full-time physicians. Gerardo had foresight. He is always on the forefront of trying to help the family doctor become more efficient when handling electronic health records.

This compilation of dot phrases is another example of his hard work, dedication and desire to help us have work-life balance, so we have time to have dinner with our families or even play golf.

Pamela Davis, MD
Program Director, Dignity Health Family Medicine Residency at
Northridge Hospital, Northridge, California

PREFACE

Early in my career I became frustrated by the additional time I spent completing my clinic notes. During residency I was baffled when my associate residency director treated patients in the hospital in the morning, treated patients in clinic in the afternoon, and in between handled administrative responsibilities. I was amazed he was able to leave the office at five (sometimes earlier to go play golf).

I noticed that all his notes were completed by the time he left the clinic. When I asked him how he did it, he showed me some templates he used that were part of the Electronic Health Record (EHR) system. They were clunky and not user-friendly, but the templates gave me an idea. Every time I found myself writing the same thing over and over, I took extra time to write a boilerplate template for that condition.

After six years I accumulated more than 1,000 boilerplate templates that I now use regularly in my practice. I typically leave the clinic on time after I have completed my notes. Although I don't play golf, I do have time for dinner with my family every evening.

This book was written to make medical documentation more efficient and help physicians avoid burnout. The dot phrases help you document office visits and procedures. They facilitate billing by providing the required documentation and simplifying billing codes. They also help you manage your inbox by providing personalized template messages for patient labs and imaging results.

I hope you find these templates useful, and they enable you to have a more sustainable work-life balance. My goal is to help physicians, residents and other healthcare providers spend more time with their patients and less time in front of the computer.

Gerardo Guerra Bonilla, MD

INTRODUCTION

The templates found in StatNote were designed for the primary-care setting. They range from documentation needed for typical visits for hypertension and diabetes to templates with documentation needed for procedures, billing and coding, face-to-face documentation for durable medical equipment (DME), and other conditions that are not as common. Toward the end of this book, there is a section of patient message templates that helps communicate lab and imaging results.

These templates are located in the phrase library and can be purchased at statnote.com. The phrase file works with a third-party text expander software that can be used with any EHR system. This book will help familiarize you with all the templates available.

A dot phrase abbreviation or description is provided at the top of each boiler template. You might change the wording to descriptive abbreviations that work for you and that are easy to recall. If you use most of the 1,000 templates, it is almost impossible to remember the description name of each one.

I find it useful to keep the dot phrases lower cased. That way it doesn't interrupt the flow of my writing. I also save some time by avoiding switching to all caps. (i.e. using ,.HTN vs ,.htn).

All the dot phrases start with a comma and a dot (,.). This should help avoid triggering your EHR's autotexts/smartphrases vs. StatNote templates.

Dot phrase suffixes and prefixes

Most conditions have two dot phrases: one that pertains to the history of present illness (HPI), or subjective part of the note, and one that pertains to the assessment and plan (A/P) part of the note (i.e ,.htn-hpi, and ,.htn#). The dot phrase for the A/P part usually has # as a suffix. The -hpi suffix is generally used for only short acronyms like HTN or AK.

Some dot phrases have a -PE suffix for the physical exam section (i.e. acne,

acne-PE and acne#).

Some conditions have up to five different templates. (i.e. „.carpal-tunnel, „.carpal-tunnel-PE, „.carpal-tunnel#, „.carpal-tunnel-inj, „.carpal-tunnel*). Note how the -hpi suffix was not used in this case.

	Dot phrase suffix and prefix legend
-hpi	subjective
-PE	objective/physical exam
-#	assessment/plan
-inj	injection - procedure documentation
-proc	procedure documentation
-*	CPT codes
em-	E/M visit codes
lab-	lab results messages
xray- or us-	imaging results messages

Some dot phrases are used as only documentation for billing purposes. For example, with transitional care management for hospital follow-ups („.hospital f/u-transitional), providers must document that the patient was contacted within two business days.

The templates have concise and relevant information regarding the different conditions being documented. You should always edit the templates in order to document accurately. For some complex patient presentations, it is better to dictate or write the old-fashioned way. Finally, you should always read your notes before you sign them.

statnote dot phrases - primary care phrase library

1 GENERAL MEDICINE

,.advance-care-planning

Advance care planning
Explained and discussed planning of medical care in the event of loss of decision-making abilities.
Discussed and filled-out Advance Healthcare Directive form.
Discussed and filled-out POLST form.
Face-to-face voluntary discussion for 16 minutes were spent during this encounter.
Present for discussion: patient only.

,.chronic-bzd

Chronic use of benzodiazepines
Indication: _
Hours able to sleep w/ med: _
Hours able to sleep w/o med: _
Symptoms reduction w/ med: _%
Taking medication as directed.
Including: alprazolam
Psychosomatic symptoms including anxiety, depression and insomnia are being treated.

Denies any side effects from medication including sedation.
Medications are not interfering with ADLs.
Addiction 4C: Denies craving, compulsive behavior, lack of self-control.
Denies negative consequences as a result of using controlled substances.
Not taking any opioids.
Does not mix with alcohol.

,.chronic-bzd#

Chronic use of benzodiazepines
Medications providing over 30% improvement of
Severity of panic attacks.
Hours of sleep.
Daily function.
No change in management. Using lowest effective dose.
Discussed alternative pharmacological and non-pharmacological therapies.
No suspected aberrant drug-taking behaviors.

,.chronic-pain

Chronic pain
Location: _
Pain w/o med: _/10
Pain w/ med: _/10
Taking medication as directed.
Including: hydrocodone, Tylenol, NSAIDs
Psychosomatic symptoms including depression and insomnia are being treated.
Denies any side effects from medication including sedation and constipation.
Medications are not interfering with ADLs.
Addiction 4C: Denies craving, compulsive behavior, lack of self-control.
Denies negative consequences as a result of using controlled substances.

,.chronic-pain#

\# Chronic pain
Medications providing over 30% improvement of pain and function.
< 90 MME.
No change in management. Using lowest effective dose.
Discussed alternative pharmacological and non-pharmacological pain relief therapies.
No suspected aberrant drug-taking behaviors.

,.cures

Cures report consistent with controlled substance agreement.
Toxicology screen via urine up-to-date.
Controlled substance agreement signed.
Not suspicious for misuse of controlled medications.

,.diet-counseling

\# Diet/exercise counseling
Counseled the patient on healthy diet and physical activity due to obesity, hypertension, diabetes, hyperlipidemia for 15 minutes.

,.fall-elderly

Pt c/o mechanical fall.
Tripped and lost balance.
Denies gait or balance impairment.
No muscle weakness.
No dementia or cognitive impairment.
No peripheral neuropathy.
Denies any dizziness or lightheadedness.
No new medications.
Environmental hazards: no loose rugs, poor lighting, clutter.

,.fall-elderly#

Fall
Recommended use of a cane or a walker.
Reviewed medications. No modifications.
Vision assessment. Consider ophtho referral.
Recommended exercise for strength and balance training (tai-chi).
Consider home safety assessment.

,.fatigue

Pt c/o fatigue x_ mo.
No SOB, CP, palpitations.
No menorrhagia.
No melena or blood in the stool.
Does not skip meals.
Sleeps >6 hours.
Not overworked.
No stress.

,.fatigue#

Fatigue
History and physical exam do not suggest any organic illness associated with fatigue.
No side effects of medications or substance misuse.
No psychiatric issues.
Good sleep quality/quantity.
Sent pt for lab w/u.

,.hospital f/u-transitional

Transitional care management. Patient was contacted within 2 business days of discharge. See note below for documentation.

,.hospital-f/u

Here for hospital discharge follow-up.
Pertinent laboratories were reviewed.
Discharge records were reviewed.
In summary _

,.marijuana

Patient reports using marijuana.
Using it for medical reasons.
Does not use more than one drug at a time.
Pt is able to stop using drug whenever wanted.
Does not report "blackouts or flashbacks" as a result of drug use.
Patient does not feel bad or guilty about drug use.
Family has not complained about involvement with drugs.
Denies any withdrawal symptoms.
Denies any medical problems as a result of drug use.

,.marijuana#

Marijuana use
DAST-10 score: 0
No problems related to drug abuse. Suggested action: None at this time.
Structured screening/Counseling on adverse effects of cannabis use.
Recommended cessation or cut down - 15 min.
1–2 Low level problems related to drug abuse. Suggested action: Monitor, re-assess at a later date.
3–5 Moderate level problems related to drug abuse. Suggested action: Further investigation.
6–8 Substantial level problems related to drug abuse. Suggested action:Intensive assessment.
9–10 Severe level problems related to drug abuse. Suggested action: Intensive assessment.

,.morbid-obesity

Morbid Obesity
Diet: high carbs.
Sugary drinks: occasional.
Etoh: occasional.
Sedentary lifestyle.

,.morbid-obesity#

Morbid Obesity
Discussed appropriate BMI.
Goal of losing 1 lb per month.
Diet modification.
Physical activity.
Encouraged/praised to build confidence.

,.naloxone

Naloxone rx sent. Concurrent use of opiates with benzodiazepines.

A prescription for naloxone intranasal kit was sent to the patient's pharmacy. Patient was educated on when and how to administer naloxone intranasal. Patient was provided with our clinic handout on naloxone administration. I have also advised the patient to share this information with friends, family, and other members of their household and offered patient the option to help train any said individuals if they so desire.

,.obesity

Obesity
Diet: high carbs.
Sugary drinks: occasional.
Etoh: occasional.
Sedentary lifestyle.

,.obesity#

\# Obesity
Discussed appropriate BMI.
Goal of losing 1 lb per month.
Diet modification.
Physical activity.
Encouraged/praised to build confidence.

,.opioids

Combined use of opioids and benzodiazepines increases the risk of extreme sleepiness, respiratory depression, coma and death. Please avoid using them at the same time. Patient expressed understanding.

,.osa-screen

OSA screen
Pt snores loudly +
Feels tired, fatigued, or sleepy during daytime +
Observed stop breathing during sleep +
H/o HTN +
BMI >35 +
Age >50 +
Neck circumference >16" +
Male +

,.osa-screen#

\# Snoring, OSA screen
STOP BANG score _
High risk of OSA (5-8)
Intermediate risk of OSA (3-4)

Low risk of OSA (0-2)
Referred to sleep medicine for sleep study.

,.overweight

Overweight
Diet: high carbs.
Sugary drinks: occasional.
Etoh: occasional.
Sedentary lifestyle.

,.overweight#

\# Overweight
Discussed appropriate BMI.
Goal of losing 1 lb per month.
Diet modification.
Physical activity.
Encouraged/praised to build confidence.

,.preop#

Preop eval
Presently Clinically Stable for Scheduled Surgery.
Avoidance of Aspirin or NSAIDS 5-7 days prior to surgery.
To call with any changes in present status.
EKG: NSR, no significant issues noted.
Labs: sent for routine preop labs and CXR.
No contraindication to surgery if normal laboratory and imaging studies.

,.preop-eval

Here for pre-op eval.
Surgeon:

Date Of Surgery:
Diagnosis:
Procedure:
No complications from previous anesthesia.
Pt has no active cardiac conditions.
No h/o CAD or prior MI.
No h/o CHF.
No h/o DM, insulin dependent.
No h/o CKD on HD.
Good functional status. Pt is able to walk four blocks or climb two flights of stairs.
Patient denies CP, SOB, or palpitations during the last six months.

,.stable

Stable. No changes in management.

,.tobacco#

Tobacco use
Counseled on smoking cessation for 3 minutes.
Readiness to quit: not interested.
Discussed treatment options with nicotine replacement.
Discussed available resources like 1-800-NO-BUTTS.

,.tobacco*

99406

,.transition-of-care

I have reviewed the discharge summary and other pertinent hospital records.
The patient does not have any pending diagnostic tests or treatments.

No problems or coordination of care issues have been identified today. Medication reconciliation has been completed during today's visit.

,.transitional-care14*

99495

,.transitional-care7*

99496

,.traveler-advice

Traveling to _
Duration: _
Not visiting relatives/friends.
Not staying with locals.
No chronic conditions.

,.traveler-advice#

Traveler advice
Discussed preventive measures.
Vaccines given.
Rx malaria ppx.

1.1 BILLING CODES

	office visit new	office visit established
low	99202	99213
mod	99203	99214
high	99204	99215

	prev med, initial (physical)	prev med, established (physical)
<1	99381	99391
1-4	99382	99392
5-11	99383	99393
12-17	99384	99394
18-39	99385	99395
40-64	99386	99396
65+	99387	99397

	annual wellness, initial	annual wellness, subsequent
medicare	G0438	G0439

	14d/MC	7d/HC
transitional care	99495	99496

	30	30+
ACP	99497	99498

	counsel	psychotherapy
tobacco	99406	90833
etoh/substance	99408	postop f/u visit
prev med	99411	99024

MC: moderate complexity
HC: high complexity

,.em+well

Outside of the Annual Wellness/Preventive Medicine E&M Visit, 10 minutes were spent face-to-face with the patient, over 50% of which was spent in counseling regarding the above problems.

,.em-office-new-low

99202

,.em-office-new-mod

99203

,.em-office-new-high

99204

,.em-office-estab-low
99213

,.em-office-estab-mod
99214

,.em-office-estab-high
99215

,.em-physical-ini-1
99381

,.em-physical-ini-1-4
99382

,.em-physical-ini-5-11
99383

,.em-physical-ini-12-17
99384

,.em-physical-ini-18-39
99385

,.em-physical-ini-40-64
99386

,.em-physical-ini-65+
99387

,.em-physical-estab-1
99391

,.em-physical-estab-1-4
99392

,.em-physical-estab-5-11
99393

,.em-physical-estab-12-17
99394

,.em-physical-estab-18-39
99395

,.em-physical-estab-40-64
99396

,.em-physical-estab-65+

99397

,.em-wellness-ini

G0438

,.em-wellness-subs

G0439

,.em-transitional-14/MC

99495

,.em-transitional-7/HC

99496

1.2 HEALTH MAINTENANCE/PHYSICALS

For Well Child Checks see Pediatrics section.

This section includes wellness Medicare visits and "physicals." The templates, with the prefix "physical-*," are categorized by age and gender. I use this template in the HPI section of the office visit note while I use the template "health-maintenance" in the A/P section.

Health Maintenance
These templates are based on current U.S. Preventive Services Task Force guidelines as well as the Centers for Disease Control and Prevention guidelines for vaccines. The templates are organized by age, gender and risk factors.

,.health-maintenance-F18+

\# Health Maintenance

(<24) Sexually active, STD/HIV screening: sent for labs.

(>18) Depression screen: denies feeling depressed or having little pleasure in doing things.

Female

(<50) Contraception: not interested.

(21-65) Cervical cancer screening: up-to-date, last pap-smear <3 yrs ago - normal.

Vaccines

Tdap: up-to-date.

Influenza vaccine: advised to get vaccine during influenza season Oct-May.

(>65, 19-65 DM/COPD,Ast/CHF) Pneumonia vaccine: n/a.

Smoker

Tobacco use: counseling on cessation.

Counseled on healthy diet and physical activity

,.health-maintenance-F25+

Health Maintenance

(>18) Depression screen: denies feeling depressed or having little pleasure in doing things.

(>35) Lipid disorders screening: up-to-date. Not on statins, 10-yr ASCVD risk <7.5%.

Female

(<50) Contraception: not interested.

(21-65) Cervical cancer screening: up-to-date, last pap-smear <3 yrs ago - normal.

Vaccines

Tdap: up-to-date.

Influenza vaccine: advised to get vaccine during influenza season Oct-May.

(>65, 19-65 DM/COPD,Ast/CHF) Pneumonia vaccine: n/a.

Smoker

Tobacco use: counseling on cessation.

Counseled on healthy diet and physical activity.

,.health-maintenance-F50+

Health Maintenance

(>18) Depression screen: denies feeling depressed or having little pleasure in doing things.

(>35) Lipid disorders screening: up-to-date. Not on statins, 10-yr ASCVD risk <7.5%.

(45/55-79) Aspirin to prevent CVD: not taking aspirin. ASCVD <10%.

(51-71) Hepatitis screening: sent, born between 1945-1965.

(50-75) Colorectal cancer screening: up-to-date.

Female

(21-65) Cervical cancer screening: up-to-date, last pap-smear <3 yrs ago - normal.

(50-74) Breast cancer screening: up-to-date, last mammogram on <2 yrs ago - normal.

Vaccines

Tdap: up-to-date.

Influenza vaccine: advised to get vaccine during influenza season Oct-May.

(>65, 19-65 DM/COPD,Ast/CHF) Pneumonia vaccine: n/a.

Smoker

(55-80) Lung cancer screening: Pt has a 30 pack-year smoking history and currently smokes or quit <15 yrs ago.

Tobacco use: counseling on cessation.

Counseled on healthy diet and physical activity.

,.health-maintenance-F60+

Health Maintenance

(>18) Depression screen: denies feeling depressed or having little pleasure in doing things.

(>35) Lipid disorders screening: up-to-date. Not on statins, 10-yr ASCVD risk <7.5%.

(45/55-79) Aspirin to prevent CVD: not taking aspirin. ASCVD <10%.

(51-71) Hepatitis screening: sent, born between 1945-1965.

(50-75) Colorectal cancer screening: up-to-date.

Female

(21-65) Cervical cancer screening: up-to-date, last pap-smear <3 yrs ago - normal.

(50-74) Breast cancer screening: up-to-date, last mammogram on <2 yrs ago - normal.

Vaccines

Tdap: up-to-date.

Influenza vaccine: advised to get vaccine during influenza season Oct-May.

(>60) Zoster vaccine: rx sent.

(>65, 19-65 DM/COPD,Ast/CHF) Pneumonia vaccine: up-to-date.

Smoker

(55-80) Lung cancer screening: Pt has a 30 pack-year smoking history and currently smokes or quit <15 yrs ago.

Tobacco use: counseling on cessation.

Counseled on healthy diet and physical activity

(60) ACP

,.health-maintenance-F65+

Health Maintenance

(>18) Depression screen: denies feeling depressed or having little pleasure in doing things.

(>35) Lipid disorders screening: up-to-date. Not on statins, 10-yr ASCVD risk <7.5%.

(45/55-79) Aspirin to prevent CVD: not taking aspirin. ASCVD <10%.

(51-71) Hepatitis screening: sent, born between 1945-1965.

(50-75) Colorectal cancer screening: up-to-date.

(>65) Fall prevention: At increased risk of falls. On vitamin D.

(>65) Osteoporosis: Not at risk. Not a smoker or daily alcohol use, BMI>21, no family history.

Female

(50-74) Breast cancer screening: up-to-date, last mammogram on <2 yrs ago - normal.

Vaccines

Tdap: up-to-date.

Influenza vaccine: advised to get vaccine during influenza season Oct-May.

(>60) Zoster vaccine: rx sent.

(>65, 19-65 DM/COPD,Ast/CHF) Pneumonia vaccine: up-to-date.

Smoker

(55-80) Lung cancer screening: Pt has a 30 pack-yr smoking history and currently smokes or quit <15 yrs ago.

Tobacco use: counseling on cessation.

Counseled on healthy diet and physical activity

(60) ACP

,.health-maintenance-M18+

Health Maintenance

(<24) Sexually active, STD/HIV screening: sent for labs.

(>18) Depression screen: denies feeling depressed or having little pleasure in doing things.

Vaccines

Tdap: up-to-date.

Influenza vaccine: advised to get vaccine during influenza season Oct-May.

(>65, 19-65 DM/COPD,Ast/CHF) Pneumonia vaccine: N/A.

Smoker

Tobacco use: counseling on cessation.

Counseled on healthy diet and physical activity

,.health-maintenance-M25+

Health Maintenance

(>18) Depression screen: denies feeling depressed or having little pleasure in doing things.

(>35) Lipid disorders screening: up-to-date. Not on statins, 10-yr ASCVD risk <7.5%.

Vaccines

Tdap: up-to-date.

Influenza vaccine: advised to get vaccine during influenza season Oct-May.

(>65, 19-65 DM/COPD,Ast/CHF) Pneumonia vaccine: N/A.

Smoker

Tobacco use: counseling on cessation.

Counseled on healthy diet and physical activity.

,.health-maintenance-M50+

Health Maintenance

(>18) Depression screen: denies feeling depressed or having little pleasure in doing things.

(>35) Lipid disorders screening: up-to-date. Not on statins, 10-yr ASCVD risk <7.5%.

(45/55-79) Aspirin to prevent CVD: not taking aspirin. ASCVD <10%.

(51-71) Hepatitis screening: sent, born between 1945-1965.

(50-75) Colorectal cancer screening: up-to-date.

Vaccines

Tdap: up-to-date.

Influenza vaccine: advised to get vaccine during influenza season Oct-May.

(>65, 19-65 DM/COPD,Ast/CHF) Pneumonia vaccine: N/A

Smoker

(55-80) Lung cancer screening: Pt has a 30 pack-year smoking history and currently smokes or quit <15 yrs ago.

Tobacco use: counseling on cessation.

Counseled on healthy diet and physical activity.

,.health-maintenance-M60+

Health Maintenance

(>18) Depression screen: denies feeling depressed or having little pleasure in doing things.

(>35) Lipid disorders screening: up-to-date. Not on statins, 10-yr ASCVD risk <7.5%.

(45/55-79) Aspirin to prevent CVD: not taking aspirin. ASCVD <10%.

(51-71) Hepatitis screening: sent, born between 1945-1965.

(50-75) Colorectal cancer screening: up-to-date.

Vaccines

Tdap: up-to-date.

Influenza vaccine: advised to get vaccine during influenza season Oct-May.

(>60) Zoster vaccine: rx sent.

(>65, 19-65 DM/COPD,Ast/CHF) Pneumonia vaccine: up-to-date.

Smoker

(55-80) Lung cancer screening: Pt has a 30 pack-year smoking history and currently smokes or quit <15 yrs ago.

Tobacco use: counseling on cessation.

Counseled on healthy diet and physical activity.

(60) ACP

,.health-maintenance-M65+

Health Maintenance

(>18) Depression screen: denies feeling depressed or having little pleasure in doing things.

(>35) Lipid disorders screening: up-to-date. Not on statins, 10-yr ASCVD risk <7.5%.

(45/55-79) Aspirin to prevent CVD: not taking aspirin. ASCVD <10%.

(51-71) Hepatitis screening: sent, born between 1945-1965.

(50-75) Colorectal cancer screening: up-to-date.

(>65) Fall prevention: At increased risk of falls. On vitamin D.

(>65) Osteoporosis: Not at risk. Not a smoker or daily alcohol use, BMI>21, no family history.

Vaccines

Tdap: up-to-date.

Influenza vaccine: advised to get vaccine during influenza season Oct-May.

(>60) Zoster vaccine: rx sent.

(>65, 19-65 DM/COPD,Ast/CHF) Pneumonia vaccine: up-to-date.

Smoker

(55-80) Lung cancer screening: Pt has a 30 pack-year smoking history and currently smokes or quit <15 yrs ago.

(65-75 M) AAA screening: up-to-date.

Tobacco use: counseling on cessation.

Counseled on healthy diet and physical activity

(60) ACP

,,physical

Here for Annual Preventive Physical Exam / Establish care.

Date of last physical: over 1 year.

Patient does not smoke.
EtOH: occasional. Not worried/guilty about drinking habits.
No drug abuse.
Diet: regular.
Exercise: regularly.
Occupation: _.
Lives at home.

No family history of diabetes, hypertension, cardiovascular disease, cancer.

Problem List

,.physical-F

Here for Annual Preventive Physical Exam / Establish care.

Date of last physical: over 1 year.

Patient does not smoke.
EtOH: occasional. Not worried/guilty about drinking habits.
No drug abuse.
Diet: regular.
Exercise: regularly.
Occupation: _.
Lives at home.
No family history of diabetes, hypertension, cardiovascular disease, cancer.

Well woman exam
Pt has never had any abnormal pap smears.
Her last pap smear was > 3 yrs ago.
Pt is sexually active w/ only one partner.
Contraception used: none.
Not interested in GC/Chlam testing.
Denies any intimate partner violence.
Pt denies any abnormal vaginal bleeding or any vaginal d/c.
Pt is regular and denies any metromenorrhagia.
Denies any breast masses or abnormalities on self-breast exam.

Problem List

,.physical-F>50

Here for Annual Preventive Physical Exam / Establish care.

Date of last physical: over 1 year.

Patient does not smoke.
EtOH: occasional. Not worried/guilty about drinking habits.
No drug abuse.
Diet: regular.
Exercise: regularly.
Occupation: _.
Lives at home.
No family history of diabetes, hypertension, cardiovascular disease, cancer.

Well woman exam
Pt has never had any abnormal pap smears.
Her last pap smear was >3 yrs ago.
Pt is sexually active w/ only one partner.
Denies any intimate partner violence.
Menopausic.
Pt denies any abnormal vaginal bleeding or any vaginal d/c.
Denies any breast masses or abnormalities on self-breast exam.

Problem List

,.wellness-exam

Here for Senior Assessment/yearly wellness exam.

Date of last physical: over 1 year.

Current healthcare providers/suppliers:

Denies feeling depressed or having little interest in doing things.
Denies sleep changes, loss of interest, guilt, lack of energy, reduced cognition or difficulty concentrating, change in appetite, psychomotor changes, suicide ideation.
PHQ-9 Score:

Functional ability/safety
Hearing: _ normal.
ADL's: Independent.

No impairment for bed mobility, transfers, ambulation, dressing, eating, or toileting and personal hygiene.
_ Requires setup help only. One person physical assistant.
Fall risk: _ no recent falls.
Home safety: feels safe at home.

Patient does not smoke.
EtOH: occasional. Not worried/guilty about drinking habits.
No drug abuse.
Diet: regular.
Exercise: regularly.
Occupation: _.
Lives at home.
No family history of diabetes, hypertension, cardiac disease, cancer.

Problem List

,.wwc#

Well Woman Check
Pelvic exam was unremarkable.
Pap smear done.
Sent specimen for GC and chlamydia.
Breast exam within normal limits.
No family history of breast cancer. Menstrual cycle is regular.
No concerns with sexual life or intimate partner violence.
Contraception: not interested.
Pt is up-to-date w/ all her immunizations.
Preventive counseling: Diet and exercise reviewed.

,.wwc-hpi

Well woman exam
Pt has never had any abnormal pap smears.
Her last pap smear was > 3 yrs ago.
Pt is sexually active w/ only one partner.
Contraception used: none.

Not interested in GC/Chlam testing.
Denies any intimate partner violence.
Pt denies any abnormal vaginal bleeding or any vaginal d/c.
Pt is regular and denies any metromenorrhagia.
Denies any breast masses or abnormalities on self-breast exam.

1.3 PHYSICAL EXAM

These templates (abdomen, ent, cardiopulm) are categorized based on the organ system pertinent to the visit. When I listen to the patient's heart and lungs, I use the cardiopulm template. The main template I use is "no-touch" (everything documented can be gathered from entering the room, saying hi to the patient and shaking his or her hand.) This template covers nine organ systems or elements required to be documented for billing purposes. I often start with the "no-touch" template and then add elements of the physical exam pertinent to the visit. You will see multiple templates in other sections with the suffix -PE (i.e. ,.acne-PE, ,.knee-PE).

,.pe-adult-xshort-(no-touch)

General: No acute distress. Awake and conversant.
Eyes: Normal conjunctiva, anicteric. Round symmetric pupils.
ENT: Hearing grossly intact. No nasal discharge.
Neck: Neck is supple. No masses or thyromegaly.
Respiratory: Respirations are non-labored. No wheezing.
Skin: Warm. No rashes or ulcers.
Psych: Alert and oriented. Cooperative, Appropriate mood and affect, Normal judgment.
CV: No lower extremity edema.
MSK: Normal ambulation. No clubbing or cyanosis.
Neuro: Sensation and CN II-XII grossly normal.

,.pe-abdomen

General: No acute distress. Awake and conversant.
Eyes: Normal conjunctiva, anicteric. Round symmetric pupils.
ENT: Hearing grossly intact. No nasal discharge.
Neck: Neck is supple. No masses or thyromegaly.
Respiratory: Respirations are non-labored. No wheezing.
Abdomen: Soft, non-tender, non-distended.
Skin: Warm. No rashes or ulcers.

Psych: Alert and oriented. Cooperative, Appropriate mood and affect, Normal judgment.
CV: No lower extremity edema.
MSK: Normal ambulation. No clubbing or cyanosis.
Neuro: Sensation and CN II-XII grossly normal.

,.pe-adult-cardiopulm

General: No acute distress. Awake and conversant.
Eyes: Normal conjunctiva, anicteric. Round symmetric pupils.
ENT: Hearing grossly intact. No nasal discharge. Oral mucosa is moist.
Neck: Neck is supple. No masses or thyromegaly.
Respiratory: Respirations are non-labored. Lungs are clear to auscultation.
Skin: Warm. No rashes or ulcers.
Psych: Alert and oriented. Cooperative, Appropriate mood and affect, Normal judgment.
CV: Normal heart sounds, no murmurs. No lower extremity edema.
MSK: Normal ambulation. No clubbing or cyanosis.
Neuro: Sensation and CN II-XII grossly normal.

,.pe-ent

General: No acute distress. Awake and conversant.
Eyes: Normal conjunctiva, anicteric. Round symmetric pupils.
ENT: Hearing grossly intact. No nasal discharge.
Clear tympanic membranes bilateral.
Pharyngeal erythema.
Neck: Neck is supple. No masses or thyromegaly.
Respiratory: Respirations are non-labored. No wheezing.
Skin: Warm. No rashes or ulcers.
Psych: Alert and oriented. Cooperative, Appropriate mood and affect, Normal judgment.
CV: No lower extremity edema.
MSK: Normal ambulation. No clubbing or cyanosis.
Neuro: Sensation and CN II-XII grossly normal.

,.breast-PE

Breasts:
No chest deformity, asymmetry. Normal contours.
_Right breast: No dimpling, no breast tenderness, nodules or masses. No axillary adenopathy. No nipple discharge.
_Right breast: _1x1 cm mass palpated at _3 OC, _4 cm from nipple. No nipple discharge. No axillary adenopathy.

,.pelvic-PE

Pelvic exam:
Labia: No erythema, No excoriation, No lesion.
Vagina: No bleeding, No discharge, No laceration.
Cervix: Os (Closed), No cervical motion tenderness, No discharge.
Uterus: Mobile, Not tender.
Ovaries: Not tender.

,.rectal-PE

Rectal: normal sphincter tone, no anal, perineal or rectal lesions, prostate is not tender, enlarged or nodular.

,.testicular-PE

GU: Genital exam revealed normal uncircumcised penis. No penile lesions or penile discharge.
No scrotal edema or tenderness, no masses.

2 CARDIOLOGY

,.afib

Atrial fibrillation
On chronic anticoagulation.
And rate control medications.
Compliant. No side effects.
Denies palpitations, CP, SOB.

,.afib#

Atrial fibrillation
Stable.
Rate controlled.
Continue anticoagulation.
No changes in management.

,.as-hpi

Aortic stenosis
Compliant with meds.
No exertional dyspnea, chest pain or syncope.

,.as#

Aortic stenosis
Asymptomatic.
Vmax < 4 m/s.
Mean pressure gradient < 40 mmHg.
Continue conservative management w/ BB, ACEi, diuretics.
Optimal BP control.
Recent stress test. 2d echo done <1 yr ago.
No CAD, CHF. EF >50%.

,.cad-hpi

CAD
Compliant with medical management and lifestyle changes.
On ASA, BB, ACE inhibitor, statin. Plavix.
Denies side effects from medications.
Denies chest pain or palpitations. Not using NTG.
No changes in exertion tolerance.
Patient does not smoke.
Not seen recently by cardiologist.

,.cad#

CAD
Stable. No changes in medical management.
Encouraged healthy lifestyle modifications.
F/u with cardiology.

,.chf-hpi

CHF
Patient is able to perform routine and desired activities of daily living.
Denies CP, palpitations, SOB, orthopnea, leg swelling.

Comfortable at rest.
Watching diet and sodium intake.
Not using tobacco, alcohol, or illegal drugs.
No recent exacerbations.
Not part of home telemonitoring program.
Not followed by cardiology.

,.chf#
=======

\# HFrEF HFpEF
NYHA I-no lim II-sx w nl activity, III-sx w minimal activity IV-sx at rest.
a - no CAD. No sx/lim activity.
b - min CAD. Mild sx/lim activity.
c - mod CAD. Comft only at rest.
c - severe CAD. Sx at rest.

LVEF <40% - on ACEi, BB.
Cautious use of diuretics.
DM, HTN, afib optimization of medical management.
Wt, edema check.
F/u w/ cardiology
 telemonitoring/ multidisciplinary ds management program.
No anemia/Fe def.

AICD candidate
LVEF < 35%, ischemic cardiomyopathy, NYHA II/III despite optimal medical rx for >3 mo.
>1 yr expected survival and good functional status.

CRT
QRS >120 ms.

,.cp-hpi
========

Pt c/o chest pain x wks.
Pain located on right side.

No radiation.
Described as pressure.
Lasts for a few minutes.
At rest. Not related to exertion.
No SOB or palpitations.
No emotional stressors.

,.cp-atypical#

Atypical chest pain
EKG w/o any acute ischemic findings.
No risk factors.
Reassured pt.
Consider stress test if persistent.

,.hld-hpi

Hyperlipidemia
Compliant with statin. No side effects.
Following a low-cholesterol diet.

,.hld#

Hyperlipidemia
Stable. Continue with current management without changes.
Discussed healthy diet and lifestyle.

,.htn-hpi

Hypertension
On _. Compliant with medications. Does not report any headaches, blurry vision, dizziness, chest pain, shortness of breath, or palpitations.
Following a low salt diet. Exercising.

,.htn#

HTN
Not Controlled.
Continue current medications. No change in management.
Discussed DASH diet and dietary sodium restrictions.
Continue/Increase dietary efforts and physical activity.

,.le-edema

C/o lower extremity edema, bilateral.
Some pain and discomfort.
High salt in diet.
No h/o CHF or CKD.
No SOB or orthopnea.
No new or changes in medications.

,.le-edema#

LE edema
Normal renal fx.
Gravity dependent.
Gecrease Na in diet.
Leg elevation and compression stockings recommended.

,.orthostatic-hypotension#

Orthostatic hypotension
Recommended adequate hydration, compression stockings, sitting before standing.

,.pad#

peripheral artery ds

Anti platelet therapy.
Statins.
Exercise.
Optimal control of cardiovascular risk factors.
ABI < 0.8 - imaging and consider vascular sx referral.

,.pad-hpi

Pt c/o intermittent claudication.
Reports leg pain with walking that is relieved with rest.

,.pvd#

peripheral artery ds
Anti platelet therapy.
Statins.
Exercise.
Optimal control of cardiovascular risk factors.
ABI < 0.8 - imaging and consider vascular sx referral.

,.pvd-hpi

Pt c/o intermittent claudication.
Reports leg pain with walking that is relieved with rest.

,.score-ASCVD

10-year ASCVD calculated risk score <5%. No need for statins.

3 DERMATOLOGY

,.accutane#

Discussed
Remember not to give your medication to anyone else. Do not donate blood. Make sure you complete your comprehension questions on ipledge and pick up your medication within 7 days or you may end up being delayed in your treatment.

,.accutane#F

Discussed
Maintain 2 forms of birth control or abstinence as discussed with your provider (during treatment and a month after). Remember not to give your medication to anyone else. Do not donate blood. Make sure you complete your comprehension questions on ipledge and pick up your medication within 7 days or you may end up being delayed in your treatment. Pregnancy test a month after the last dose.

,.acne

Pt c/o facial acne.

Using topicals w/o significant improvement.
No scars.
Not affecting chest or back.

,.acne#

Acne
BPO wash.
Clindamycin gel.
Topical retinoid.

,.acne-PE

Open/closed comedones and erythematous papules and pustules. No nodules/cysts. No pitted/hypertrophic scars. Face/upper trunk involved.

,.acne-baby

Multiple inflammatory papules, small pustules/closed comedones at cheeks w/ some erythematous background.

,.acne-sx-comedo*

10040

,.ak-hpi

Patient complains of scaly lesion on _.
Present for many months.
C/o some itching.
No personal or family history of skin cancer.
+ sun exposure. Does not use photoprotection.

,.ak#

Actinic keratosis
Cryotherapy done.
Discussed photoprotection.

,.ak-PE

Scaly and rough papule with ill-defined borders on

,.alopecia-female

Alopecia
Complains of hair loss for the last few months.
Endorses family history of baldness.
Reports diffuse thinning of the central scalp with preservation of frontotemporal hairline.

,.alopecia-male

Alopecia
Complains of hair loss for the last few months.
Endorses family history of baldness.
Reports gradual receding of frontal hairline and crown.

,.alopecia#female

Alopecia, female pattern
Negative hair-pull test.
Lab w/u: TSH, iron panel, CBC, fee testosterone, and RPR.
Trial of minoxidil, topical.

Consider spironolactone if not improving.

„.alopecia#male

Alopecia, androgenic
Negative hair-pull test.
Lab w/u: TSH, iron panel, CBC, fee testosterone, and RPR.
Trial of minoxidil, topical.
Consider finasteride if not improving.

„.alopecia-areata

Pt c/o patch of hair loss on scalp.
Reports some emotional stress lately.
No itching or burning sensation in the area.
No h/o atopic dermatitis, vitiligo or thyroid ds.

„.alopecia-areata-PE

Round, patchy areas of nonscarring hair loss on occipital area measuring 3 x 3 cm. Also affecting right cheek 1 x 1 cm. No hypopigmentation areas. Exclamation point Hairs observed.

„.alopecia-areata-inj*

11900

„.alopecia-areata-inj

Intralesional steroid injection.
After discussion of risks and benefits of corticosteroid injection, including but not limited to infection, bleeding, discomfort with injection, skin atrophy or color changes, injury to surrounding structures, elevated blood

sugar, and possibility of no improvement, patient gave verbal and written consent.
Area was cleaned with alcohol.
1 cc of Kenalog 4 mg/mL mix with plain 1% lidocaine were injected on _left occipital area.

,.alopecia-female-PE

Marked reduction in terminal hair density present on bitemporal and occipital area.

,.alopecia-male-PE

Marked reduction in terminal hair density present on the frontal hairline and vertex.

,.bedbug-PE

Urticaria-like papules and vesicles on exposed areas (neck, arms, hands). linear configuration.

,.bedbug#

Bedbug bite
Eradication of infestation discussed with patient.
Prn oral antihistamines and topical steroids.

,.cheilitis

C/o dry and burning pain on lips.
Reports some redness.
Does not improve with chapstick.
Denies lip licking.

".cheilitis#

Cheilitis, eczematous
Vaseline use.
Short course of triamcinolone.
Avoid lip licking.

".cheilitis-PE

Erythematous lips with some scaling, no fissures.

".claravis#

Discussed
Remember not to give your medication to anyone else. Do not donate blood. Make sure you complete your comprehension questions on ipledge and pick up your medication within 7 days or you may end up being delayed in your treatment.

".claravis#F

Discussed
Maintain 2 forms of birth control or abstinence as discussed with your provider (during treatment and a month after). Remember not to give your medication to anyone else. Do not donate blood. Make sure you complete your comprehension questions on ipledge and pick up your medication within 7 days or you may end up being delayed in your treatment. Pregnancy test a month after the last dose.

,..cradle-cap

Mother brings infant w/ c/o crusty scales on scalp.
No other areas of the body affected.
No other rash. No fever. Otherwise healthy and feeding well.

,..cradle-cap#

Cradle cap
Education, reassurance, conservative management.
Emollients and frequent shampooing to soften and remove scales.
Consider ketoconazole shampoo if not improving. (2x/wk x 2wks).

,..cradle-cap-PE

Well-defined, erythematous macules and plaques w/ greasy, yellow scale involving frontal scalp and cheeks.

,..cryotherapy*1-AK

17000

,..cryotherapy*2-14-AK

17003

,..cryotherapy-AK

Cryotherapy
Consent: Risks and benefits of therapy discussed with patient who voices understanding and agrees with planned care. No barriers to communication or understanding identified.

After obtaining informed consent, the patient's identity, procedure, and site were verified during a pause prior to proceeding with the minor surgical procedure as per universal protocol recommendations.
_ Actinic keratosis on _ treated with light cryotherapy using cryocautery with freeze thaw freeze technique with 2-3 mm surround freeze.
No complications. Procedure was well tolerated.

,.cryotherapy-SK

Cryotherapy
Consent: Risks and benefits of therapy discussed with patient who voices understanding and agrees with planned care. No barriers to communication or understanding identified.
After obtaining informed consent, the patient's identity, procedure, and site were verified during a pause prior to proceeding with the minor surgical procedure as per universal protocol recommendations.
_ Seborrheic keratosis lesions on _ treated with light cryotherapy using cryocautery with freeze thaw freeze technique with 2-3 mm surround freeze.
No complications. Procedure was well tolerated.

,.cryotherapy-wart

Cryotherapy
Consent: Risks and benefits of therapy discussed with patient who voices understanding and agrees with planned care. No barriers to communication or understanding identified.
After obtaining informed consent, the patient's identity, procedure, and site were verified during a pause prior to proceeding with the minor surgical procedure as per universal protocol recommendations.
_ Warts on _ treated with light cryotherapy using cryocautery with freeze thaw freeze technique with 2-3 mm surround freeze.
No complications. Procedure was well tolerated.

,..cryotherapy-wart*1-14

17110

,..cryotherapy-wart*15

17111

,..cryotherapy-wart-plantar

Cryotherapy
Consent: Risks and benefits of therapy discussed with patient who voices understanding and agrees with planned care. No barriers to communication or understanding identified.
After obtaining informed consent, the patient's identity, procedure, and site were verified during a pause prior to proceeding with the minor surgical procedure as per universal protocol recommendations.
Wart was treated with shave excision of overlying keratin and then cryocauterized with freeze thaw freeze technique with 2-3 mm surround freeze.
No complications. Procedure was well tolerated.

,..dermatofibroma

Pt c/o bump on skin present for years.
Located on leg.
Does not recall any trauma or insect bite.
Denies any pain or itchiness.
No irritation with shaving.

,..dermatofibroma#

Dermatofibroma
Reassurance. Monitor.

Recommended occlusive dressing at night.
Trim nails, wear gloves at night.
Currently no evidence of superimposed infection.
Liberal use of emollients (vaseline, moisturizer).
Discouraged prolonged use of topical corticosteroid d/t skin atrophy.
Avoid hot water.
Loratadine and benadryl prn itching. Topical benadryl.
Return if condition worsens or fails to improve.
Consider dermatology and/or allergist referral if no improvement.

,.eczema-PE

Erythematous plaques on extensor arms, evidence of excoriation.

,.folliculitis

Pt c/o red bumps on trunk and buttocks.
Recent use of a hot tub.
Does not shave the area.
No new drugs.

,.folliculitis#

Folliculitis
Reassured. Usually self limited.
Wash with antibacterial soap. Topical mupirocin.
Prevent recurrence with BPO wash.
Cool, dry, loose clothing.
Consider po meds if recurrent/severe.

,.folliculitis-PE

Multiple follicular erythematous papules/pustules on _

,.folliculitis-scalp

Pt c/o red bumps on the back of neck.
Using topicals w/o significant improvement.
pt uses razor/trimmer to shave head.

,.folliculitis-scalp#

Folliculitis, scalp/neck
Avoid shaving/trimming.
Trial of BPO wash and topical mupirocin.

,.fragile-nails

Pt c/o fragile nails and brittleness.
Household daily chores are particularly damaging.
Denies any fatigue or h/o anemia.

,.fragile-nails#

Onychorrhexis
Recommended nail varnish.
Avoid humidity/prolonged exposure to water.

,.fragile-nails-PE

Longitudinal nail grooves with distal splits affecting all nails.

,.granuloma-annulare

Hand: annular nonscaly reddish-brown plaque. Plaque centers are hypopigmented relative to the edges.

,.granuloma-annulare#

Granuloma annulare
Localized disease.
Trial of topical steroids.
Consider intralesional steroid injection or cryotherapy if not improving.

,.herpes-labialis

Pt c/o painful sore on lip.
Present for days.
Reports tingling sensation around lesion.
Denies any fevers.
No other lesions.

,.herpes-labialis#

Herpes labialis
Po valacyclovir 2g bid x1d.
+ topical antiviral, docosanol 10%.
Symptomatic tx w/ nsaids/tylenol, topical lidocaine.

,.herpes-labialis-PE

Single ulcer along the vermillion border on left upper lip.

,.hyperhidrosis

Pt c/o of excessive palmar and plantar sweating.
Started when she was young.
No severe facial, axillary or generalized sweating.

,.hyperhidrosis#

Hyperhidrosis
Trial of topical aluminum chloride.

,.hyperhidrosis-PE

Excess sweat noted bilaterally on the palms of the hands.

,.impetigo#

Impetigo
Contact precautions.
Localized - topical mupirocin.
Widespread - po abx (cephalexin).

,.impetigo-PE

"Honey-crusted" plaques with small inflammatory halos.

,.intralesion-inj*

11900

,.intralesion-injection

Intralesional steroid injection.
After consent was obtained.
Area was cleaned with betadine.
0.25 mL of Kenalog 40 mg/mL was injected on lesion _

,.keloid-injection

Intralesional steroid injection
After consent was obtained.
Area was cleaned with betadine.
0.25 mL of Kenalog 40 mg/mL was injected on keloid scar on left ear lobule.

,.keloid-scar

Pt c/o slowly growing scar on _.
Inciting event: body piercing, surgery.
No itchiness, tingling or pain.

,.keloid-scar#

Keloid scar
Silicone-based therapy.
Consider intralesional corticosteroid injection.

,.keloid-scar-PE

Smooth and shiny elevated scar with overhanging edge on _.

,.lichen-planus-PE

Purple planar patch on _

,.lichen-planus#

Lichen planus
Clobetasol topical, taper down as soon as improving.

,.onychomycosis

Patient complains of changes in toenails for years.
Reports thickening and discoloration of toenails.
Denies any toenail trauma.
Tried OTC treatment without improvement.

,.onychomycosis#

Onychomycosis
Confirmed diagnosis with microscopic test.
Start terbinafine.
Send patient for liver function tests.

,.onychomycosis#f/u

Onychomycosis
Did not achieve complete resolution with po meds. Trial of topical ciclopirox.

,.onychomycosis-PE

Multiple toenails with marked nail thickening, yellowish nail discoloration, onycholysis, and subungual debris.

,.paronychia

Paronychia
Patient c/o pain, tenderness, and swelling in lateral fold of nail of _

,.paronychia#

Paronychia

With abscess. Incision and drainage performed.
Started amoxicillin/clavulanate 875/125 po bid.
Daily wound care.

,.paronychia*

10060

,.paronychia-PE

_ erythema and pus surrounding nail fold. Tender and fluctuant to palpation.

,.paronychia-proc

Paronychia with abscess I&D
Location: right _
Consent obtained.
Local anesthesia achieved with ethyl chloride. Area cleaned with alcohol.
Puncture incision made with 18 G needle inserted under the affected cuticle margin. Small amount of white thick material was expressed.
Hemostasis achieved with compression.
Wound dressed with dry, sterile dressing. Pt tolerated procedure well.

,.penile-sebaceous-h

Pt c/o whitish lesion on scrotum and penis.
No new sexual contacts.
No dysuria or penile discharge.
Lesion is not painful.
Present for months.

,.penile-sebaceous-h#

Penile sebaceous hyperplasia
Reassured pt.
Consider cryotherapy if bothersome.

,.penile-sebaceous-h-PE

Smooth white colored papules on shaft of penis and scrotum. not tender to palpation.

,.psoriasis

C/o white spots on skin.
Present for several months.
Affecting trunk and scalp.
Denies any nail involvement or joint pain.

,.psoriasis#

Psoriasis
Moderate, affecting >3% body surface area.
Affecting nails.
Started topical treatment.
Clobetasol and triamcinolone for intertriginous areas.
Calcipotriene.
Neutrogena T/Sal shampoo.
Consider systemic tx. Referral to rheumatology.

,.psoriasis-PE

Sharply demarcated erythematous, silver scale plaques of the scalp, elbows and knees, neck/chest.
Axillae and groin also involved.

Nail pitting observed.

,.punch-bx

Punch Biopsy of _Left leg lesion.
Skin cleaned with 70% alcohol swab.
Area anesthetized with 1% Lidocaine without epi.
Area was prepped in usual sterile fashion with 10% Iodine swab and sterile drapes, and sterile gloves used.
Using a _5 mm circular Punch device, downward pressure was applied to obtain a cylindrical core of tissue.
Tissue specimen removed easily with Iris scissors and Adson forceps.
Wound closed w/ 4-0 Nylon suture. 2 simple interrupted sutures placed.
Hemostasis achieved.
Triple antibiotic ointment and bandaid applied.
Specimen sent to pathology.

,.punch-bx-1*

11104

,.punch-bx-2+*

11105

,.rash

C/o rash
Involving face, scalp ,mouth, trunk, extremities, diaper area, flexure area.
Has been present for days, worsening.
Spread to _ from initial area.
Not pruritic.
Not associated w/ fever, arthralgias, URI symptoms, or other recent viral syndromes.

Interventions to date: OTC hydrocortisone cream, non responsive.
Precipitating factors:
No new medications.
Denies any insect bites.

,.rosacea

Rosacea
C/o redness and flushing of central face.
Worsens with certain foods.
No ocular involvement.

,.rosacea#

Rosacea
Trial of metronidazole topical.
Consider po doxycycline if not improving.

,.rosacea-PE

Erythema of central face, including cheeks, nose, and central forehead. + telangiectasias.

,.scabies#

Scabies
Rx permethrin x2.
Advised tx for all members of household.
Instructed pt on decontamination of linens, clothing, furniture, etc.
Short course tx w/ hydrocortisone.
Benadryl prn itching.
Liberal use of emollients.

,.scabies-PE

Multiple burrows along erythematous papules on elbows, around umbilicus, lower abdomen, upper and lower extremities. Head and neck spared. excoriations 2/2 scratching.

,.seborrheic-dermatitis

Seborrheic dermatitis
C/o itching and scaling on glabella, scalp, nasolabial fold.
Reports some redness.

,.seborrheic-dermatitis#

Seborrheic dermatitis
Short-term course of topical steroids.
Daily use of clotrimazole

,.seborrheic-dermatitis-PE

Loose, greasy scales within erythematous, fine patches involving forehead, nasolabial folds and chin.

,.senile-purpura

Pt c/o bilateral hand bruising.
Not on anticoagulant.
No h/o trauma.

,.senile-purpura-PE

Multiple purpuric macule and patches on bilateral dorsal hands and extensor forearms.

,.senile-purpura#

Senile purpura
Minimize trauma to skin as possible (wear layer of clothing to protect arms).
Sun avoidance/photoprotection.
Reassurance. Self-limited condition.
Avoid aspirin.
Consider topical amlactin solution for dry skin.

,.shave-bx

Shave Biopsy of _Left upper back lesion: size _
Skin cleaned with 70% alcohol swab. Area anesthetized with 1% Lidocaine. Area was prepped in usual sterile fashion with 10% Iodine swab and sterile drapes, and sterile gloves used. Lesion shaved off with Dermablade. Hemostasis achieved with drysol and direct pressure. Triple antibiotic ointment and bandaid applied. Specimen sent to pathology.

,.shave-bx* (not removal of lesion)

11102

,.shave-bx*-trunk/arm/leg <0.5 cm

11300

,.shave-bx*-trunk/arm/leg 0.6-1 cm

11301

„.shave-bx*-trunk/arm/leg 1.1-2 cm

11302

„.shave-bx*-trunk/arm/leg >2 cm

11303

„.shave-bx*-scalp/neck/hand <0.5 cm

11305

„.shave-bx*-scalp/neck/hand 0.6-1 cm

11306

„.shave-bx*-scalp/neck/hand 1.1-2 cm

11307

„.shave-bx*-scalp/neck/hand >2 cm

11308

„.shave-bx*-face <0.5 cm

11310

,.shave-bx*-face 0.6-1 cm

11311

,.shave-bx*-face 1.1-2 cm

11312

,.shave-bx*-face >2 cm

11313

,.shingles

Shingles
Pt c/o rash on _
Painful and itchy.
Present for days.

,.shingles#

Herpes zoster
Immunocompetent pt.
Mild pain.
Start po antiviral (valacyclovir 1g tidx7d).
Prn analgesics, calamine lotion.

,.shingles-PE

Grouped vesicles on an erythematous base confined to a distinct dermatome on _ without crossing the midline.

,.sk-hpi

Pt c/o lesion on _torso painless but c/o itching/irritation.
No bleeding.

,.sk#

Seborrheic keratosis
Reassured pt. Monitor.

,.sk-PE

1x1 cm "stuck-on" appearance, hyperpigmented lesion w/ wart-like texture located on face.

,.sk-irritated#

Seborrheic keratosis, irritated
Cryotherapy done.

,.skin-tag

Pt c/o skin tag located on _
Present for months.
Irritated when caught on jewelry or rubbed by clothing.

,.skin-tag#

Skin tags
Lesions removed.
Wound care at home reviewed.

,..skin-tag-PE

Pedunculated skin colored lesion on _

,..skin-tag-removal

Removal of skin tags - _bilateral neck area:
Skin cleaned with 70% alcohol swab.
_ skin tags excised easily with Iris scissors.
Hemostasis achieved with drysol and direct pressure.
Triple antibiotic ointment and bandaid applied

,..skin-tag-removal*

11200

,..solar-lentigo#

Solar lentigo
Reassured. Monitor.
Photoprotection.
Consider bx if enlarging or darkening.
Consider cryotherapy or laser if bothersome.

,..solar-lentigo-PE

1x1 cm smooth light brown pigmented macule on _

,..solar-lentigo

Pt c/o dark spot on face.
Similar lesions on dorsal hands and forearms.
+ sun exposure, no photo-protection use.

Present for months.
Not increasing in size or changing in color.

,.tinea-inguinale

Patient complains of skin lesion present on groin.
x months.
Worsening.
Itching.

,.tinea-inguinale#

Tinea inguinale
Topical antifungal therapy. Cream and powder.
Continue for a week after clearing.
Discussed perspiration management.

,.tinea-inguinale-PE

Annular, red/hyperpigmented, scaly plaques extending from the inguinal creases, down to medial thigh, and buttocks. Demarcated edges.

,.tinea-pedis

Patient complains of skin lesion present on feet.
x months.
Worsening.
Itching.

,.tinea-pedis#

Tinea pedis

Topical antifungal therapy. Cream and powder.
Continue for a week after clearing.
Discussed perspiration management.

,.tinea-pedis-PE

Bilateral plantar feet w/ white scaly skin in a "moccasin" distribution.

,.tinea-versicolor

Patient complains of skin lesion present on torso.
x months.
Worsening.
Itching.

,.tinea-versicolor#

Tinea versicolor
Po fluconazole 1x/wk x2wk. Perspire during tx days.
Topical antifungal therapy.
Continue for a couple of weeks after clearing.

,.tinea-versicolor-PE

Multiple hypopigmented macules and patches with fine bran-like scale. Lesions are oval and coalesce. Affect in chest and back. No facial involvement.

,.unna-boot*

29580

Present for months.
Not increasing in size or changing in color.

,.tinea-inguinale

Patient complains of skin lesion present on groin.
x months.
Worsening.
Itching.

,.tinea-inguinale#

Tinea inguinale
Topical antifungal therapy. Cream and powder.
Continue for a week after clearing.
Discussed perspiration management.

,.tinea-inguinale-PE

Annular, red/hyperpigmented, scaly plaques extending from the inguinal creases, down to medial thigh, and buttocks. Demarcated edges.

,.tinea-pedis

Patient complains of skin lesion present on feet.
x months.
Worsening.
Itching.

,.tinea-pedis#

Tinea pedis

Topical antifungal therapy. Cream and powder.
Continue for a week after clearing.
Discussed perspiration management.

,.tinea-pedis-PE

Bilateral plantar feet w/ white scaly skin in a "moccasin" distribution.

,.tinea-versicolor

Patient complains of skin lesion present on torso.
x months.
Worsening.
Itching.

,.tinea-versicolor#

Tinea versicolor
Po fluconazole 1x/wk x2wk. Perspire during tx days.
Topical antifungal therapy.
Continue for a couple of weeks after clearing.

,.tinea-versicolor-PE

Multiple hypopigmented macules and patches with fine bran-like scale. Lesions are oval and coalesce. Affect in chest and back. No facial involvement.

,.unna-boot*

29580

,.unna-boot-proc

Procedure: Unna boot.
Location: Right lower extremity.
A 3-inch gauze impregnated with calamine-gelatin-zinc oxide compound was used to place a unna boot compression bandage in a crisscross pattern beginning at the metatarsal-phalangeal joint and ending just below the level of the tibial tuberosity. A second layer was applied using an elastic bandage using the same pattern.
Patient tolerated procedure well. Instructed patient to keep dressing dry and to remove if there are any symptoms of impaired circulation including any paresthesia, discoloration, or worsening discomfort.

,.vitiligo

Pt c/o periorificial depigmentation.
Areas involved include: periocular, perioral, perianal/genital, and axillae.
Present for years.
Not improving.
Failed OTC tx.

,.vitiligo#

Vitiligo
Widespread, affecting >3% body surface area.
Discussed treatment options including:
  phototherapy.
  topical clobetasol or tacrolimus.

,.vitiligo-PE

Depigmented patches on axillae, perioral, periorbital.

,.wart

Pt c/o lesion growth over the last few months.
Location: _
Painful.

,.wart#

Wart
Cryotherapy done.
Salicylic acid gel.

,.wart-PE

Hyperkeratotic, skin colored papule on _

,.wart-plantar#

Plantar wart
Cryotherapy done.
Salicylic acid gel.

,.wart-plantar-PE

Left plantar foot: hyperkeratotic, skin-colored papule with tiny black dots in the lesion. overlying callus.

4 ENDOCRINOLOGY

,.acanthosis-nigricans-PE

Symmetric, dark brown hyperpigmented plaques with a velvety appearance on neck folds, axillae and inframammary folds.

,.dm2#

Diabetes Mellitus type 2
Not Controlled. Hyperglycemia.
Continue current medications. No change in management.
Patient is on aspirin, ACEI, and statin.
Lipid panel checked less than a year ago.
Microalbumin checked less than a year ago.
Foot exam and monofilament test done.
Continue/Increase dietary efforts and physical activity.
Routine diabetic retinopathy screening: up-to-date.

,.dm2-PE

Monofilament screen: normal sensation on feet. 2+ pulses. No ulcers.

,.dm2-insulin

Insulin-dependent diabetes type 2
On _ units of Lantus qhs and _ units of Humalog qac. As well as metformin.
Compliant with medications. No hypoglycemic events.
Fasting blood glucose _
Postprandial blood glucose _
No complaints of foot pain or paresthesias.
Seen by ophthalmologist: <1 yr ago.
Following a low carb diet.

,.dm2-pomed

Diabetes type 2
On metformin, glipizide
Compliant with medications. On ACEI. No hypoglycemic events.
Not checking blood glucose at home.
No complaints of foot pain or paresthesias.
Seen by ophthalmologist <1 yr ago.
Following a low carb diet. Exercising.

,.hyperthyroidism

Graves' disease
On methimazole. Compliant with medications. No side effects.
Denies heat intolerance, sweating or unintentional weight loss.
No tremors or palpitations.

,.hyperthyroidism#

Graves disease
Stable. TSH checked less than a year ago.
Continue current medications w/o change.

„.hypothyroidism

Hypothyroidism
Patient is on levothyroxine. Compliant with medication, denies any side effects like palpitations.
Denies any fatigue, weight gain, cold intolerance, constipation, or dry skin.

„.hypothyroidism#

Hypothyroidism
Stable. TSH checked less than a year ago.
Continue current medications w/o change.

„.low-testosterone

Pt c/o decreased libido, erectile dysfunction with loss of morning erections.
Denies gynecomastia, shrinking/small testes, or infertility.
Also reports fatigue and decreased energy levels.

„.low-testosterone#

Male hypogonadism
8-10 AM total testosterone.
If low (<300 ng/dL) consider repeat, including LH/FSH.
Discussed affecting factors like weight and age.

„.osteoporosis

Osteoporosis
Not taking medications.
No back pain.
Impaired gait, using a walker to ambulate.
No recent falls.

,.osteoporosis#

Osteoporosis
No h/o osteoporosis fractures, not a high-risk patient.
Recent Dexa scan T-score >-3.5.
Bisphosphonate for <5 years.
Discussed the risks/benefits of therapy.

,.vit-d-def

Pt wants to be screened for vit D deficiency.
C/o fatigue.
Denies any muscle weakness.
No h/o CKD.
Denies inadequate sunlight exposure.
Reports having a good diet, including dairy products.
No h/o IBDs, celiac, CF, or surgeries causing malabsorption.
Pt is obese.

,.vit-d-def#

vit D deficiency
No risk factors.
Check 25-OH vit D, calcium.
Consider supplementation if <20.
Discussed sun exposure, Ca/vit D diet intake.

5 ENT & OPHTHALMOLOGY

,.allergic-rhinitis

Pt c/o sneezing, nasal pruritus.
Some nasal congestion and rhinorrhea as well.
Palate, throat, ear, and eye itching.
No eye redness.

,.allergic-rhinitis#

Allergic rhinitis
Intermittent mild symptoms.
Trial of flonase, oral antihistamine, and allergen avoidance.
Consider leukotriene receptor if symptoms become persistent/moderate.

,.cataracts

Pt c/o gradual decrease in vision.
Endorses blurred or cloudy vision.
Glare when driving at night.

,.cataracts#

Cataracts
Some functional visual impairment.
Correction of refractive error.
Consider intraocular lens implant.
Referred for annual eye exam.

,.cataracts-PE

Bilateral eyes with cloudy intraocular lens.

,.cerumen-impaction

Pt c/o right ear decreased hearing and popping sensation x days.

,.cerumen-impaction#

Cerumen impaction
Ear lavage done.
Avoid use of Q-tips.

,.chalazion-PE

Upper eyelid, _left: nontender, mild erythematous firm nodule just above tarsal plate.

,.conjunctivitis

C/o bilateral watery eye discharge for months.
+ itching.
No contact lens use.
No mucoid or purulent discharge.

Eyelids not stuck together in am.
No periocular tenderness.
Some rhinorrhea, pt has allergies.

,.conjunctivitis#bacterial

\# Conjunctivitis
Counseling on good hand hygiene, no contact lens use while sx present.
Trial of cool compresses and liberal use of refrigerated artificial tears.
  Mod-severe bacterial
Rx ofloxacin 0.3% 1 gtt qid x7d.
Rx polytrim 1 gtt qid x7d.

,.conjunctivitis#viral

\# Conjunctivitis
Counseling on good hand hygiene, no contact lens use while sx present.
Trial of cool compresses and liberal use of refrigerated artificial tears.
 Viral / mild bacterial
Reassured on self-limiting condition.
Rx 0.5% erythromycin oint qid x7d.

,.conjunctivitis-allergic#acute

\# Allergic conjunctivitis
Instructed not to rub the eyes, d/c contact lens use, apply cold compresses.
Liberal use of refrigerated artificial tears.
  Acute - Short-term tx (2 wk) of opht antihistamine.
(naphazoline, ketotifen, or olopatadine 0.2% 1 gtt qd).

,.conjunctivitis-allergic#chronic

\# Allergic conjunctivitis
Instructed not to rub the eyes, d/c contact lens use, apply cold compresses.

Liberal use of refrigerated artificial tears.
Chronic - mast cell stabilizer (cromolyn 4% 2 gtt q6h) + antihistamine.

,.ear-lavage

Ear lavage
_Right ear irrigated with lukewarm water, hydrogen peroxide, and OtoClear.
Large piece of brown cerumen extracted with ear curette.
TM: wnl. Pt tolerated procedure well.

,.ear-lavage*

69210

,.ear-lavage*FOB

69200

,.ear-lavage-FOB-removal

Ear foreign body removal
Under direct visualization, foreign body from the _ external auditory canal was removed using alligator forceps.
Pt tolerated procedure well.

,.epistaxis

Pt c/o bleeding from the nose.
Recurrent with several episodes in the last few days.
No h/o bleeding disorders.
Not on anticoagulation.
Denies easy bruising or gum bleeding.

,.epistaxis#

Epistaxis, anterior
Recommended cool mist humidifier.
Nasal saline spray + vaseline.
Prn afrin.

,.epistaxis-PE

Blood oozing from nasal septum.

,.epistaxis*cauterization/pack-ant

30901

,.epistaxis-cauterization

Cauterization of epistaxis, left nasal septum
Afrin/epinephrine saturated gauze was packed into _left nasal space.
Exam of nasal membrane revealed oozing from medial septum (Kiesselbach's plexus area).
Silver nitrate was used for cauterization.
Patient tolerated procedure well.
Bacitracin was applied afterwards.
No need for expandable nasal sponge.

,.eustachian-tube-dys

Patient complains of right ear pain, sensation of ear fullness.
Some hearing loss.
Recent URI.
No history of allergies.

,.eustachian-tube-dys#

\# Eustachian tube dysfunction
Trial of decongestants and nasal steroids.
Yawning/Swallowing.
Toynbee maneuver.

,.glaucoma

Glaucoma
On opt gtt.
Compliant.
Denies any loss of peripheral vision or eye pain.

,.glaucoma#

\# Glaucoma
Stable. Continue opt gtt.
Monitor intraocular pressure and symptoms like vision changes, redness or eye pain.

,.hearing-loss

Pt c/o gradually progressive hearing loss.
C/o difficulty understanding words/conversation in a busy/noisy environment.
No history of noise exposure.

,.hearing-loss#conductive

\# Gradual CHL
Likely cerumen impaction. - ear lavage done.
Eustachian tube dysfunction - trial of decongestant.
Consider audiology evaluation.

,.hearing-loss#presbycusis

\# Gradual SNHL
Most likely presbycusis.
Referred to audiology.
Consider amplification w/ hearing aids.
Discussed cost and infrequent insurance coverage.
Listening strategies: lip reading, direct facing, slow speaking.

,.hearing-loss#sudden

\# Sudden hearing loss
Referral to ENT.

,.hearing-loss-PE

Bilateral ear exam
Normal auricle.
No mastoid tenderness.
Normal ear canal and tympanic membrane.
Normal drum mobility using pneumatic otoscopy.
Negative whisper test (repeats 6/6 words).
Weber - symmetric (forehead).
   lateralizes to _ (blocked ear in CHL, better ear in SNHL.
Rinne - normal (air > bone conduction) (mastoid).
   negative (bone > air conduction) (CHL).

,.mucocele

Mucocele
Pt c/o painless cyst on lower lip.
Present for weeks. Increasing in size.
No h/o mouth trauma.

,.mucocele#

Mucocele
Of lower lip.
Drainage and cryotherapy done.
Postprocedure care: pressure for the next hour.
Topical antibiotic ointment to avoid irritation/infection.
Pain control as needed with OTC meds.
Healing expected within 1-2 wks.

,.mucocele*cryo

40820

,.mucocele*drain

40810

,.mucocele-PE

Left lower lip: 7x7 mm nontender, mobile, dome-shaped enlargement with intact epithelium that lies over it. Translucent.

,.mucocele-proc

Procedure: Mucocele destruction
Indication: Lower lip mucocele.
Consent: A consent form was signed and witnessed after a discussion with the patient/guardian of the risks (including but not limited to pain, bleeding, infection, scar formation, slow healing, recurrence of lesion, and failure to diagnose more serious pathology), benefits (treatment of lesion),

and alternatives (including but not limited to simple aspiration, excision, and watchful waiting).

Technique: The mucosa surrounding the lesion was cleansed with Betadine and then anesthetized with lidocaine 1% with epinephrine 1 : 100,000 through a 30-gauge needle, using a total volume of 3 mL. Anesthesia was confirmed. A small stab wound was made in the cyst laterally using an 11 blade, and the seromucinous contents were expressed.

The lesion was frozen with liquid nitrogen with a 2-mm rim of normal tissue included for 5 seconds. Final hemostasis was achieved with brief application of electrocautery to any visible areas of bleeding. Antibiotic ointment was applied to the lesion.

Complications: None
Estimated blood loss: Less than 5 mL
Follow-up: If needed for any signs or symptoms of infection or recurrence of lesion.

,.otitis

C/o _ ear pain x days.
No fever or chills.
Denies any otorrhea.
No headache, pain over mastoid area, neck pain or photophobia
No recent URI sx or sinus infx
No h/o previous OM.

,.otitis#

Acute otitis media
Tylenol prn pain or fever
Rx amoxicillin 500 mg PO tid x 7d
Return if no improvement after 48-72 hrs

,.otitis#viral

Acute otitis media
Likely viral
Pt is afebrile, mild discomfort
Tylenol prn pain or fever
Return if fever, otorrhea, worsening or no improvement after 48-72 hrs

,.otitis-externa#

Otitis externa
Start Ciprodex.
NSAIDs for pain control.

,.otitis-externa-PE

Right ear with external canal edema and purulence. + tragal tenderness. No mastoid tenderness.

,.pterygium

Pterygium
Pt c/o ocular irritation, burning and tearing
Noticed conjunctival lesion on _right eye.
Hx of chronic UV light exposure.
Denies any blurred vision or any other vision disturbance.

,.pterygium#

Pterygium
Bilateral.
Causing irritation. - trial of artificial tears.
Not causing visual impairment.
UV light protection.

Consider referral to ophthalmology if not improving.

,.pterygium-PE

Eyes, bilateral: wing-shaped conjunctival overgrowth onto the corneal surface. Nasal side. Not crossing the midline.

,.sialadenitis

Pt c/o of facial swelling and pain.
No dysphagia.
Similar previous episode.
No fever or chills.
Denies any pus coming from salivary gland opening.
Not taking anticholinergic medications.

,.sialadenitis#

Sialadenitis
Recurrent (<3x/yr).
No infection.
Conservative management.
Hydration, pain relief, and sialogogues.
Suck lemon/tart candies. Massage and milk the duct.
Refer to ENT if not improving with conservative management or recurring.

,.sialadenitis-PE

Right cheek: edematous, tender to palpation, no exudates from salivary gland opening.

,.red-eye

C/o _ red eye x days
Denies decreased vision or foreign body sensation.
+ mild, burning pain. sandy/gritty feeling in the eye.
+ URI sx's.
No periocular tenderness
Endorses mild purulent/watery d/c.
Eyelids stuck together in am.
+ itching. pt has h/o allergies.
No contact lens use.

,.stye

Pt c/o _ upper eyelid lesion present for wks.
Some pain and discomfort.
Not affecting vision.
No purulence.
No fever or chills.

,.stye#-Chalazion (Chillnopain)

Chalazion
W/o significant surrounding cellulitis - amoxi/clav 500
Not distorting vision. - refer to ophtho.
Topical erythromycin.
Warm compresses + massage with diluted baby shampoo.

,.stye#-Hordeolum (Hurts)

Hordeolum
W/o significant surrounding cellulitis - amoxi/clav 500
Not distorting vision. - refer to ophtho.
Topical erythromycin.
Warm compresses + massage with diluted baby shampoo.

,.stye-PE-chalazion

Right upper eyelid swelling and erythema with a painless, rubbery, nodular lesion.

,.stye-PE-hordeolum

Right upper eyelid: tender, mild erythematous firm nodule just above tarsal plate.

,.subconjunctival-hemorrhage

Pt c/o bright red patch on _left eye x days.
Painless, no denies any trauma.
Reports coughing, rubbing eye.
Denies any vision problems.
Not using any anticoagulants.

,.subconjunctival-hemorrhage#

Subconjunctival hemorrhage
Reassurance.
Expect resolution in a couple of weeks.

,.subconjunctival-hemorrhage-PE

Left eye: extravasated blood on conjunctiva.

,.thrush

Pt c/o white painful lesion on oral mucosa/tongue.
Tried to scrape but pain persists.

,.thrush#

Oral candidiasis/ thrush
Topical antifungal.
Aggressive disinfection of removable dentures.

,.thrush-PE

Creamy white plaque fairly adherent to oral mucosa/tongue.

,.tinnitus

Pt c/o episodic pulsatile sounds for the last few months.
Denies any hearing loss or dizziness.
Denies hx of noise exposure.
Denies visual changes.

,.tinnitus#

Tinnitus
Troublesome.
Not affecting quality of life.
Education and counseling.
Consider CBT.

6 GASTROENTEROLOGY

,.asplenia#

\# Asplenia
Menactra given.
Rx meningococcal B.
Pneumovax given.
Bactrim prn fever.

,.celiac-ds

Pt c/o abdominal discomfort, diarrhea and bloating.
Symptoms seem to improve when following a gluten-free diet.
No family hx of Celiac ds or IBD.
Denies any fatigue, wt loss, rashes.

,.celiac-ds#

\# Gastrointestinal symptoms suggestive of Celiac ds
Serologic testing (tTG/IgA) while pt is on a gluten-containing diet.
If positive will sent to GI for endoscopy.

,..constipation

Patient complains of constipation.
Some straining/hard stools.
Bowel movements - not daily.

,..constipation#

Constipation
Trial of MiraLax.
Once pt has regular bowel movements start diet w/ high fiber content.
Plenty of fluids.
Return if symptoms fail to improve or worsen

,..crohn-ds

Crohn's disease
On _. Compliant. No side effects.
Denies any abdominal pain, diarrhea, or blood in the stools.
No recent flares.
No arthropathies, cutaneous or ocular manifestations.

,..crohn-ds#

Crohn's disease
Stable. No recent flares.
Continue current management.
Monitor CBC/CMP, vit B12 def.
Not on chronic corticosteroids.
Colonoscopy up-to-date.
Avoid NSAIDs.
Recommended high-fiber diet.

,.gerd

GERD
C/o heartburn/regurgitation.
Denies cough, shortness of breath, sore throat, changes of taste.
No dysphagia.
No chest pain.

,.gerd#

GERD
Empiric low-dose PPI tx x 8 wks.
Maintenance and prn tx w/ H2RA afterwards.
No suspected reflux complications (Barret/stricture).
Lifestyle modification: wt loss, avoid meals 2-3h before bedtime.
Consider eliminating food triggers: chocolate, caffeine, EtOH, acid/spicy food.

,.ibs-hpi

Patient complains of abdominal discomfort. Described as crampy.
Located in the lower/mid abdomen. Can be mild to severe.
Endorses alteration of bowel habits associated with pain.
Alternating diarrhea and constipation. Relief of pain with defecation.
+ Bloating. Improved with passage of flatus.
No nausea or vomiting.

,.ibs#constipation

Irritable bowel syndrome
Constipation predominant.
 With pain or bloating.
Discussed dietary modifications. Behavioral changes, decrease stress.
Decrease caffeine, lactose and fructose.
Increase fiber intake in diet.

Consider probiotics.
Trial of MiraLAX.
Dicyclomine 10 mg qid prn spasms.
Consider SSRI, CBT.

,.ibs#diarrhea

\# Irritable bowel syndrome
Diarrhea predominant.
Loperamide prn diarrhea.
Discussed dietary modifications. Behavioral changes, decrease stress.
Decrease caffeine, lactose and fructose.
Increase fiber intake in diet.
Consider probiotics.
Dicyclomine 10 mg qid prn spasms.
Consider SSRI, CBT.

,.lactose-intol

Pt c/o symptoms of abdominal pain, flatulence, and bloating after consuming dairy products.
No diarrhea.

,.lactose-intol#

\# Lactose intolerance
Limit dairy products.
Consider lactase supplements.
Consider monitoring vit D if dairy intake is eliminated.

,.ulcerative-colitis

Ulcerative colitis
On _. Compliant. No side effects.

Denies any abdominal pain, diarrhea, or blood in the stools.
No recent flares.
No arthropathies, cutaneous or ocular manifestations.

,.ulcerative-colitis#

Ulcerative colitis
Stable. No recent flares.
Continue current management.
Monitor CBC/CMP, vit B12 def.
Not on chronic corticosteroids.
Colonoscopy up-to-date.
Avoid NSAIDs.
Recommended high-fiber diet.

7 HEMATOLOGY/ONCOLOGY

,.anemia

Anemia
Pt c/o fatigue.
No SOB, CP, palpitations.
No melena or blood in the stool.

,.anemia#Fe

Anemia, iron deficiency
Continue iron supplementation/iron-rich diet.
Asymptomatic.

,.anemia#AOCD

AOCD
Asymptomatic.
Monitor.
Treatment of underlying disease.

,.lymphadenopathy

Pt c/o lump.
Located on the neck, right.
x wks.
Denies any recent infections or URI symptoms.
Denies occupational exposures.
Does not have pets.
No recent travel or high-risk behaviors.
Denies any fever, night sweats, or unexplained weight loss.

,.lymphadenopathy#

Lymphadenopathy, cervical ,right
Young pt (<50).
< 4 weeks , < 1 cm, localized.
Reassure, low-risk of malignancy.
If persisting for over a month or increasing in size consider work up.
No need for bx at this point.

,.lymphadenopathy-PE

1x1 cm nodular, non-tender, mobile mass on right cervical area.

8 INFECTIOUS DISEASES

,.cellulitis

Pt c/o redness on skin.
Location: _
Present for days.
Became painful, redness worsening.
No spontaneous drainage.
No fever or chills.
No h/o trauma or injury.
No history of bug bite.

,.cellulitis#

Cellulitis
>2 cm surrounding erythema.
w/o pus - trial of Cephalexin or Dicloxacillin.
possible bite, anaerobic coverage - trial of amoxicillin/clavulanate (Augmentin).
Procedure precautions discussed with patient, including fever or worsening of purulent discharge.

,.cellulitis#mild

Cellulitis, mild
Trial of mupirocin.

,.cellulitis#pus

Cellulitis
>2 cm surrounding erythema.
w/ pus - trial of PO Clindamycin or TMP/SMX (Bactrim).
possible bite, anaerobic coverage - trial of amoxicillin/clavulanate (Augmentin).
Procedure precautions discussed with patient, including fever or worsening of purulent discharge.

,.cellulitis-PE

Macular erythema with indistinct borders on _. Warm and tender to touch. No fluctuance.

,.dental-clearance

Here for dental clearance.
Will undergo a dental procedure that involve manipulation of gingival tissue/periapical region of teeth or perforation of oral mucosa (including routine dental cleaning).
Not taking anticoagulants.
Pt has no prosthetic heart valves.
No h/o infectious endocarditis.
No h/o repaired congenital heart ds w/ residual shunts or valvular regurgitation.
No recent repair of congenital heart defects.
No h/o transplanted heart w/ valve regurgitations.

,,.dental-clearance#

\# Dental clearance
Cleared for dental procedure.
Pt is not high risk for infective endocarditis.
No antibiotic prophylaxis required.
According to the American Heart Association antibiotic prophylaxis with dental procedures is reasonable for patients with cardiac conditions associated with the highest risk of adverse outcomes from endocarditis.
Amoxicillin 2g 60 min prior to the dental procedure.

,,.hepC

Hepatitis C
No h/o IV drug use.
No h/o transfusion or organ transplantation.
Denies constitutional symptoms.
No jaundice, ascites, or symptoms of hepatic encephalopathy.
Has not been treated.
Interested in treatment.

,,.hepC#

\# Hepatitis C
No cirrhosis. Eval liver enzymes.
Treatment naive. Interested in treatment.
Recheck viral load.
Referral to GI.

,,.herpes-genital

Pt c/o painful sore on genitals.
Present for days.
Reports tingling sensation around lesion.
Denies any fevers.

No dysuria.
Recurrent episode.

,.herpes-genital-recurrent

Pt c/o painful sore on genitals.
Present for days.
Reports tingling sensation around lesion.
Denies any fevers.
No dysuria.
New sexual contact.

,.herpes-genital-PE

Multiple tender genital lesions, vesicles/crusted papules.

,.herpes-genital#

Genital herpes
First episode.
Valacyclovir 1000 bid x7d.
Symptomatic tx of pain (po/topical).
Screen for other STDs.

,.herpes-genital#recurrent

Genital herpes
Recurrent.
Valacyclovir 500 bid x3d.
Symptomatic tx of pain (po/topical).

,.hiv-hpi

HIV
On antiretrovirals. Compliant. No side effects.
No recent respiratory, GI, or skin infections.
No recent hospitalizations.
+ neuropathy. Feet pain controlled.

,.hiv#

HIV
Stable. On antiretroviral therapy.
Optimal CD4 count. No need for prophylactic for opportunistic infections.
Neuropathy stable.

,.prep

Pt with risky sexual behavior.
Interested in pre-exposure prophylaxis for HIV.
No h/o HIV infection.

,.prep#

High-risk sex behavior
Start PrEP with Truvada.
Monitor adherence.
HIV/STD test q3mo.
Discussed safe sex.
Check BMP.
No risk factors for renal ds. No UA needed.

,.prep#on-demand

High-risk sex behavior

Start HIV on-demand PrEP.
Safe-sex.
Check and monitor renal fx, HIV/STD.
Discussed PrEP on-demand is not FDA approved.
It is taken 2 to 24 hours prior to sexual activity, one tablet is then taken daily while sexually active, and then continued for two more days after sexual activity has stopped.

,.std-hpi

New sexual partner.
Desires to be screened for STDs.
Denies any dysuria or penile discharge.
No genital lesions.

,.std#

STD
Ceftriaxone IM 250 mg x1 given.
Rx Azithromycin 1 g x1.
Abstain from sexual activity x1 wk.
Notify partners with sexual contact in the last 60 days.
Consider Expedited Partner Therapy (EPT).

,.tb-clear

Record of Latent Tuberculosis Treatment Completion

The following is a record of evaluation and treatment for latent tuberculosis infection:

- Tuberculin Skin Test (TST):
 Date:_ Results (in millimeters of induration):_

- IGRA:

Date:_ Type of test: Gold quantiferon. Result: positive.

- Chest radiograph:
Date:_ Results: normal.

- Date medication started:_. Date completed:_.
Medication(s):_

This person is not infectious. Patient may always have a positive TB skin test, so there is no reason to repeat the test. If you need any further information, please contact my office.

,.tb-latent

Latent TB
+ PPD/gold quant.
Not pregnant, HIV uninfected.
CXR was unremarkable.
No heavy alcohol use.
Pt denies cough, fever, night sweats, weight loss or any other constitutional symptoms.
Not taking warfarin, contraceptives, antiarrhythmics.

,.tb-latent#

Latent TB
+ PPD/gold quant.
Not pregnant, HIV uninfected. Low-Incidence setting.
r/o active TB: neg CXR, asymptomatic, no need for AFB sputum.
monotherapy with rifampin x4 mo (10mg/kg, max600).
monotherapy with isoniazid x6 mo (5mg/kg, max300).
 Pyridoxine supplementation (25mg).
Baseline liver enzyme testing.
Monthly monitoring for hepatitis.
Discussed symptoms including anorexia, N/V, dark urine, ictericia, RUQ pain.

,.tb-screen

Patient here for tuberculosis screening.
No history of previous positive PPD.
Denies being an immigrant from a high tuberculosis incidence country (Mexico, Philippines, Vietnam, India, China, Haiti, and Guatemala).
Denies any close or casual contacts with active pulmonary/respiratory TB.
Patient is not a healthcare worker nor has other occupations in which there is risk of exposure to patients with untreated contagious active TB (prison facilities, homeless shelters).
Patient denies having HIV infection.
Does not have a history of transplant, chemotherapy, or other major immunocompromising condition.
Patient denies having history of abnormal chest radiographs.
Patient does not take immunosuppressive medications or undergoing dialysis.
No history of diabetes or use of chronic glucocorticoids.
Not a cigarette smoker.
Denies any chronic cough or constitutional symptoms.

,.tb-screen#

TB screening
Patient is at low-risk for developing tuberculosis.
She would not benefit from TB treatment, therefore further testing is not indicated.
However patient desires to volunteer at school and PPD testing is mandatory.
PPD given.
Return in 48 hours for reading.

9 NEUROLOGY

,.alzheimer

Alzheimers dementia
+ memory loss and disorientations.
Difficulty naming objects/people.
Misplacement of items.
Getting lost.
Apathy.
Decline in activities of daily living.
Reports:
Anxiety
Insomnia

,.alzheimer#

Alzheimer dementia
Stable. Continue supportive care.
Caregiver in place.
Safe environment at home.
Cholinesterase inhibitors.
No depression.
No anxiety.

No insomnia.

,.bell-palsy

Pt c/o sudden onset left facial weakness.
Normal sensation.
C/o dry eye on same side.
No fever/chills, rash, myalgia/arthralgias.
No previous similar episodes.

,.bell-palsy#

Bell palsy
No suspicion for CVA or Lyme.
Prednisone 60 mg po x7d. (Within 48 hrs).
No presumed HSV info - no antivirals rx.
Artificial tears/eye ointment, eye patch at night - prn incomplete eye closure.
Reassured complete recovery is likely.

,.bell-palsy-PE

Left face: complete ipsilateral paralysis of CN VII, including forehead.

,.cognitive-impairment

Family has concern for pt's memory, forgetfulness.
Report gradual decline.
No new medications or recent acute illness.
No h/o cardiovascular ds.
No depression.
Pt does not drive or manages finances.
No problems with language/word finding.
Not getting lost in familiar places.

No behavior problems.

,.cognitive-impairment#

Cognitive impairment, mild
Screen for B12 deficiency and hypothyroidism.
Consider neuroimaging.
Mini-mental state examination score:
No depression.

,.concussion

S/p head trauma - direct.
Transmitted to the head by the acceleration-deceleration of the body on impact.
Denies loss of consciousness.
Event was witnessed.
Denies previous head injury, brain trauma or alcohol/substance abuse.
c/o
headache
feeling foggy/slow
dizziness/balance problems
memory difficulties
nausea/vomiting

,.concussion#

Concussion, w/o LOC
No imaging needed at this point.
Normal physical neurologic exam.
No neuropsychological abnormalities.
Physical rest.
Cognitive rest.
Education + gradual return to activity plan.
Analgesia.

Return if symptoms fail to improve or worsen.

,.cva-hpi

CVA
Residual hemiparesis.
On PT/OT.
No problems with diet.
Pt compliant with anti platelet therapy and statins.
No recent falls.
Endorses depression.

,.cva#

CVA
Residual hemiparesis.
Stable.
Continue antiplatelet and statin tx.
Continue PT/OT/ST.
Optimal BP and glycemic control.
Continue management for depression.

,.dementia

Family has concern for pt's memory, forgetfulness.
Report gradual decline.
No new medications or recent acute illness.
No h/o cardiovascular ds.
No depression.
Pt does not drive or manage finances.
No problems with language/word finding.
Not getting lost in familiar places.
No behavior problems.

,.dementia#

Dementia
Screen for B12 deficiency and hypothyroidism.
Consider neuroimaging.
Mini-mental state examination score:
No depression.

,.dementia-f/u

Dementia
Caregiver reports no significant decline since last visit.
No significant changes in memory, forgetfulness.
No new medications or recent acute illness.
No depression.
Pt does not drive or manage finances.
No problems with language/word finding.
Not getting lost in familiar places.
No behavior problems.

,.dementia-f/u#

Dementia
Stable.
No depression.
Caregiver in place with good support.
Recommended physical activity/exercise.

,.dizziness

Patient complaints of dizziness for days.
Described as "the room is spinning".
Precipitated by sudden changes in position, head movement. getting up quickly.
Improved when eyes are closed.

Episodes last _seconds. >2 times a day.
Denies decreased hearing. Denies tinnitus. Denies nausea or vomiting.
Denies feeling faint. No history of syncope.
Does not take any blood pressure medications.
No history of cardiovascular disease or stroke.
No history of psychiatric conditions or migraines.
Denies any CP/SOB. Denies any numbness or weakness.
No history of trauma.
No recent URI or AOM.
No fever or rashes.
No new or changes in medications.

,.dizziness#

Dizziness
No signs or symptoms of central vertigo.
Orthostatic signs are [negative].
History and provocative maneuvers on physical exam suggest peripheral etiology.
Most likely etiology BPPV.

,.dizziness#BPPV

Benign paroxysmal positional vertigo
Patient education and reassurance.
Canalith repositioning - Epley maneuvers explained to patient, handout given to patient.
Meclizine prn.

,.dizziness#Meniere

Meniere disease
Supportive therapy.
Rx meclizine, scopolamine, mild sedative.
Salt restriction.

,.dizziness#vestibular

Acute vestibular neuritis
Supportive care.
Patient education and reassurance.

,.dizziness-PE

Ears: Bilateral TMs, clear. Normal hearing.
Eyes: PERRLA. EOMI. No nystagmus.
Cardiovascular: RRR, NL S1/S2, no murmurs.
Neurologic: CN 2-12 WNL. No dysmetria. No ataxia. Negative Romberg's.
Negative Dix-Hallpike test.
Negative Head Impulse test.
No Nystagmus.
Negative Test of Skew.

,.headache

Pt c/o headache.
Sudden/gradual onset _days ago. worsening.
Located: _. No radiation.
Described as throbbing, pounding, dull, sharp.
Pain is intermittent/constant.
Lasts for hours.
Does not awake pt from sleep.
Relieved with _
Exacerbates with _certain foods.
No aura.
No photophobia, no phonophobia.
No nausea, no vomiting.
Denies any recent emotional stress.
No previous similar episodes.
No h/o trauma.

Denies h/o migraines, cluster headaches, tension headaches.
Denies chronic use of NSAIDs or recent d/c of caffeine.
Does not smoke. denies any drug use.
No recent URI symptoms.
LMP: wks ago.

,.hiccups

Pt c/o persistent hiccups.
Started days ago.
Denies excessive alcohol or food consumption.

,.hiccups#

Hiccups, persistent
Did not improve with nasopharynx stimulation, supraorbital pressure, carotid sinus massage.
Trial of metoclopramide 5 mg tid.

,.mci#f/u

Mild cognitive impairment
Stable.
No depression.
Good community support.
Recommended physical activity/exercise.

,.mci-f/u

Mild cognitive impairment
No significant decline since last visit.
No significant changes in memory, forgetfulness.
No new medications or recent acute illness.
No depression.

Still able to manage finances.
No problems with language/word finding.
Not getting lost in familiar places.
No behavior problems.

,.migraine

Migraine headaches
Migraine episodes unchanged. On Imitrex prn.
Avoids triggers.
Effects on daily activities: decreased activity level.
Interfering w/ daily activities at school/work/home.
Interfering w/ sleep.
Associated symptoms: aura, sensitivity to light, visual disturbance, N/V.

,.migraine#

Migraine headache w/o aura
Controlled w/ abortive treatment prn.
No need for preventive treatment at this point.
Discussed trigger avoidance and behavioral modification.
(sleep, regular meals, hydrations, regular exercise).

,.ms#

Multiple sclerosis
Stable.
MRI done <1 yr ago.
Fatigue w/u: vit D/B12, thyroid.
Recommended regular exercise, sleep hygiene, and low-fat diet.
Mind-body therapy: yoga, relaxation.
Optimal control of chronic conditions.

,.ms-hpi

Multiple sclerosis
No recent relapses.
Motor symptoms: leg weakness, problems ambulating. No spasms.
Sensory symptoms: pain and dysesthesia.
No urinary symptoms.
No visual impairment.
No fatigue.
On no meds.

,.occipital-neuralgia

Pt c/o sudden onset headache that starts in the neck and radiates to the vertex area/eye.
Right sided. Described as stabbing pain with persistent aching between paroxysms.
Pain is debilitating. Minimal improvement with NSAIDs/tylenol.

,.occipital-neuralgia#

Occipital neuralgia
Recommended conservative tx.
Application of local heat/cold to alleviate muscle spasm/pain.
Consider local occipital nerve block to alleviate the pain.

,.occipital-neuralgia-inj

Occipital neuralgia injection
Location: bilateral suboccipital region.
Injection: 40 mg of triamcinolone + 1 mL of 1% lidocaine using a 25 G 1 in needle. on ea site.
Entry point was marked.
Area was prepped in the usual sterile manner.
The needle was inserted into the affected area and the steroid was injected.

Patient tolerated procedure well without complications.
Standard post-procedure care was explained and return precautions given.

,.occipital-neuralgia-inj*

64405

,.osa-on-cpap

OSA on CPAP
Good adherence to CPAP use.
Comfortable with CPAP pressures and mask fit.
Reports improvement in alertness and quality of life.

,.osa-on-cpap#

OSA on CPAP
Good compliance.
Symptoms improved.
Continue to monitor.

,.paraplegia

Paraplegic 2/2 spinal cord injury, wheelchair bound. Wife is primary caregiver.
Neurogenic bowel
Having regular bowel movements w/ current bowel regimen.
Neurogenic bladder
Self cath q6hrs.
No recent symptoms of autonomic dysreflexia.
No pressure ulcers noted by patient or caregiver.
Spasticity well control with current dose of baclofen.

,.paraplegia#

Paraplegia 2/2 spinal cord injury
Stable. Continue bowel regimen, self-cath and baclofen.
Monitor for pressure ulcers, autonomic dysreflexia.
Spasticity well controlled. Continue current dose of baclofen.

,.parkinson

Pt c/o resting tremor of upper limbs.
Rigid and slow movements.
No recent falls.
No memory problems.
No fatigue.
No depression.

,.parkinson#

Parkinson ds
Trial of carbidopa/levodopa 50 mg tid. titrate according to response.
Recommended physical activity. tai-chi.

,.parkinson-PE

Masked facies, resting tremor of upper extremities, rigidity, cogwheeling noted. Micrographia. Shuffling gait.

,.quadriplegia

Here accompanied by caregiver _.
Quadriplegia d/t spinal cord injury at _ level after _ years ago.
Pt is wheelchair bound.
Neurogenic bladder. Pt does intermittent self cath q4h. No recent UTIs.
Neurogenic bowel. Compliant with bowel regimen.

No reported episodes of autonomic dysreflexia.
No reported skin lesions.
Pt is being followed at _. By Dr. _.
No changes in management during last visit.

,.quadriplegia#

Quadriplegic 2/2 spinal cord injury after _.
Stable.
Continue self-cath and bowel regimen for neurogenic bladder/bowel.
No episodes of autonomic dysreflexia.
No skin lesions. Monitor. Continue frequent repositioning.
f/u at _.

,.rls-hpi

Pt c/o dysesthesias described as tingling, cramping and aching of the lower extremities.
Symptoms usually worsen later in the day, often in the hours preceding sleep.
Symptoms decrease momentarily with movement, stretching or massage.

,.rls#

Restless leg syndrome
Intermittent mild symptoms.
Trial of nonpharmacologic options including massage, exercise, stretching and warm bath before bedtime.
Avoid nicotine, alcohol, caffeine.
If symptoms worsen consider gabapentin.
Workup for fatigue, rule out iron deficiency anemia.

,.seizures

Seizures
Patient has had h/o seizures for years. Compliant with medications.
Last seizure _ ago. Patient has about _ seizures per month.
Patient does follow-up with neurologist. No changes in management during last visit.

,.seizures#

Seizures
Stable. Continue current medications unchanged.
Follow-up with Neurology.
Benzodiazepines at home PRN seizures.

,.spinal-cord-inj

Here accompanied by caregiver _.
Para/Quadra plegia d/t spinal cord injury at _ level after _ years ago.
Pt is wheelchair bound.
Neurogenic bladder. Pt does intermittent self cath q4h. No recent UTIs.
Neurogenic bowel. Compliant with bowel regimen.
No reported episodes of autonomic dysreflexia.
No reported skin lesions.
Pt is being followed at _. By Dr. _.
No changes in management during last visit.

,.spinal-cord-inj#

Para/Quadri plegic 2/2 spinal cord injury after _.
Stable.
Continue self-cath and bowel regimen for neurogenic bladder/bowel.
No episodes of autonomic dysreflexia.
No skin lesions. Monitor. Continue frequent repositioning.
f/u at _.

,.syncope

Syncope
Patient reports abrupt, brief, total LOC & postural tone with spontaneous recovery. Denies any postictal symptoms.
Denies prior episodes.
Situation: Pt was _ at time of event.
Provocative factors: exertion, changing position, eating, coughing, sneezing, swallowing, anxiety, pain, defecation/micturition.
Associated symptoms: Denies CP, dyspnea, palpitations.
Pt is amnestic to events.
Event was not witnessed.
Denies any recent changes in medications.
Denies family history of cardiac ds or sudden cardiac death.

,.syncope#

Syncope
Unexplained etiology, possibly vasovagal.
Reflex/neurocardiogenic syncope 2/2.
Single episode, no red flags. - Reassurance.
No suspicion for cardiac etiology. normal EKG, no hx of cardiac ds. no Need for echocardiogram at this point.
No suspicion for neurologic etiology, including seizures or CVA. no Head trauma. no need for CT head at this point.
No need for driving restrictions.
Recommended adequate hydration to avoid orthostatic hypotension.
Will check CBC and BMP to eval for anemia or any electrolyte abnormalities.
F/u in 3 months or return to clinic or ED if symptoms recur.

,.syncope-PE

General: NAD.

Orthostatic VS _normal.
HEENT: NC/AT, no evidence of tongue bites/injury. MMM.
Cardiac: Normal S1 and S2, no murmurs, RRR. No carotid bruits. No JVD.
Carotid massage: negative (no asystole or dec SBP >50 mmHg).
Pulmonary: CTAB.
Neurologic: no focal deficits.

,.tremor

Pt c/o hand tremors.
Brought out by arm movement/sustained positions.
Affecting daily activities like writing, drinking from a glass and handling eating utensils.
No head or voice involvement.
Symptoms improve with etoh consumption.
Worsens with anxiety.

,.tremor#rest/int

Essential tremors
Trial of propranolol.
Consider primidone.
Discussed side effects.
Differential
 Intentional tremors - cerebella. No dysmetria on exam.
 Tremors at rest - Parkinson. No phasies or other suggestive exam findings.

,.tremor-PE

Bilateral upper extremity tremor activated by voluntary movement/holding hands outstretched.
Tremor absent with limbs relaxed. No head or voice involvement.
No dysmetria.

10 OB/GYN

,.abnormal-vaginal-bleed

Pt c/o vaginal bleeding
Metromenorrhagia for months.
Sexually active. not associated with intercourse.
Does not use OCP or other forms of contraception.
LMP: wks ago.
Reports _regular periods q_d, lasts _d. _passing clots.
Soaked pad/tampon q_h.
Bleeding does _ occur between menstrual periods.
Menopausic, no use of HRT. Maternal menopause at age _.
No h/o OB sx or c/s.
Denies personal or fam hx of bleeding disorders.
Denies use of anticoagulants.
Pt is _ obese. no known h/o PCOS.

,.abnormal-vaginal-bleed#

Abnormal vaginal bleeding
Pregnancy was ruled-out.
Sent for CBC and TSH.
Sent for transvaginal US.

Consider endometrial biopsy.
Trial of OCPs and NSAIDs.

,.bartholin-cyst

Pt c/o a pimple/vulvar mass x days.
Reports vulval pressure or fullness.
Some pain with walking/sitting. + dyspareunia.
No fevers or chills. No spontaneous rupture.

,.bartholin-cyst#large

Bartholin gland cyst/vulvar abscess
 Large (<5 cm)
Conservative therapy w/ warm compresses and sit baths. Pain control.
I&D with word catheter placement done in the office.
Start empiric abx w/ MRSA coverage - TMP-SMX (Bactrim).

,.bartholin-cyst#small

Bartholin gland cyst/vulvar abscess
 Small (<2 cm)
Conservative therapy w/ warm compresses and sit baths.
If worsening or lesion points to the skin surface, consider I&D.
If not improving in 2 days start empiric abx - TMP-SMX (Bactrim).

,.bartholin-cyst*

56420

,.bartholin-cyst-PE

vulva: tender, fluctuant mass with surrounding erythema and edema.

,.bartholin-cyst-proc

Bartholin gland cyst/abscess I&D with word catheter placement

Informed consent was obtained. Risks and benefits discussed with patient. Patient was placed in the dorsal lithotomy position. Labia and vagina was prepped in the usual sterile manner with betadine. 3 cc of 1% lidocaine w/o epi were injected over intended site of entry. Incision made with an 11 scalpel blade immediately adjacent to the hymenal ring. Adson forceps with teeth were slid along the blade and grasped the tissue, defining a tract into the cyst. Abscess was drained completely and loculations were broken with a hemostat. Cultures were obtained. Word catheter was placed through the incision along the forceps. Balloon was inflated with 3 cc of saline. Catheter was gently tugged to ensure placement. Exposed portion of the catheter was tucked into the vagina. Patient tolerated procedure well.

,.colposcopy*

56821

,.colposcopy*w/o-bx

56820

,.colposcopy-proc

Colposcopy
After consent was obtained, speculum inserted and cervix visualized, No abnormalities noted. Green filter did not demonstrate any abnormalities. Vinegar applied, no lesions seen. Os very small, unable to use endocervical

speculum to visualize canal. Biopsies taken at _5:00, 6:00 and ecc due to lack of visual correlates to pap smear findings. Minimal bleeding easily controlled with pressure and monsel's solution. Patient tolerated procedure well. Pathology specimens sent. Patient will be notified with results.
Labia: Within normal limits.
Vagina: Within normal limits.

,.contraception

Pt requesting contraception.
Pt is on OCPs.
No h/o VTE, smoking, migraines w/ aura.

,.contraception#

Desired contraception
Discussed contraceptive means available including IUD, nuvaring, combination oral contraceptives, and nexplanon.
She wishes to proceed with _
Urine HCG obtained and is ***NEGATIVE***
Benefits and risks discussed with the patient.

,.depo

Desired contraception
Discussed contraceptive means available including IUD, nuvaring, combination oral contraceptives, and nexplanon.
She wishes to proceed with Depo-Provera injection. Patient currently not taking any birth control.
LMP: wks ago.
No PMH of diabetes, hypertension, or smoking.

,.depo#

Pregnancy test negative. Depo-provera was injected after patient signed informed consent. No complications. Benefits and risks discussed with the patient. Patient aware of amenorrhea/irregular bleeding, delayed fertility after discontinuation. Patient tolerated procedure well.
f/u in 3 months for repeat injection.

,.dysmenorrhea

Pt c/o painful menstruation.
Affecting daily activities.
No HA, fatigue, N/V.

,.dysmenorrhea#

Dysmenorrhea
Trial of NSAIDs and hormonal contraception.

,.emb#

Abnormal uterine bleeding.
Endometrial biopsy done without complications. Endometrial sample set for path, we will call patient with results when available.
Usual post procedure warnings and aftercare instructions reviewed. Patient was discharged in good condition.

,.emb*

58100

,.emb-proc

Endometrial biopsy with plastic endometrial aspirator (pipelle)
After appropriate discussion of risks and benefits written informed consent was obtained. The patient was placed in the dorsal lithotomy position. A bimanual exam revealed normal size and position of the uterus. A sterile speculum was inserted. The cervix was visualized and prepped with iodine. A tenaculum was applied to the anterior lip of the cervix. The aspirator with internal piston was inserted through the cervix and into the uterine cavity. The depth of the uterus was _8cm. Negative pressure was built up by drawing back the piston. The sheath was rotated 360 degrees while withdrawing the aspirator from the fundus up to the internal os. Four passes were completed, each time the tissue collected was expressed into the formalin bottle. The sample was sent to pathology. The patient tolerated the procedure well with no complications. Return precautions and standard post-procedure care discussed with patient.

,.hot-flashes

Patient c/o hot flashes and night sweats.
Menopausic.
Interfering with daily activities, bothersome.
Causing irritability and mood swings.

,.hot-flashes#

Menopause / hot flashes
Trial of non-hormonal therapies.
Black cohosh/soy isoflavones.
Consider paroxetine or venlafaxine.

,.infertility

Infertility

Reports inability to conceive for more than 12 months of frequent unprotected intercourse.
Regular menstrual periods.
No h/o oligo/amenorrhea.
No h/o STDs or suspected tubal disease/endometriosis.
No h/o chemo or radiotherapy.
Male partner has not undergone semen analysis.

,.infertility#

Infertility
Meets criteria - frequent unprotected sex recommended.
Semen analysis.
Ovulatory function assessment.
 OTC ovulatory prediction kit to detect LH surge.
 If progesterone <3 —> prolactin, TSH, LH/FSH r/o PCOS.
> 35 y/o - test ovarian reserve - menstrual cycle day 3 FSH and estradiol level

,.iud-proc-mirena

IUD Placement - Mirena
After appropriate discussion of risks and benefits of IUD placement, written informed consent was obtained. Urine pregnancy test was negative. A bimanual exam revealed normal size and position of the uterus. The patient was placed in the dorsal lithotomy position, and a sterile speculum was inserted. The cervix was visualized and prepped with iodine. A tenaculum was applied to the anterior lip of the cervix. A sound was placed through the cervical os in sterile fashion, and the uterus sounded to _8 cm. The IUD was loaded into the applicator in the usual fashion and the indicator placed according to the sound. The applicator was inserted into the cervix and the intrauterine device placed high in the endometrial cavity. The applicator was withdrawn and the strings trimmed. The patient tolerated the procedure well with no complications.

„.iud-proc-paragard

IUD Placement - Paragard

After appropriate discussion of risks and benefits of IUD placement, written informed consent was obtained. Urine pregnancy test was negative. A bimanual exam revealed normal size and position of the uterus. The patient was placed in the dorsal lithotomy position, and a sterile speculum was inserted. The cervix was visualized and prepped with iodine. A tenaculum was applied to the anterior lip of the cervix. A sound was placed through the cervical os in sterile fashion, and the uterus sounded to _8 cm. The IUD was loaded into the applicator in the usual fashion and the indicator placed according to the sound. The applicator was inserted into the cervix and the intrauterine device placed high in the endometrial cavity. The applicator was withdrawn and the strings trimmed. The patient tolerated the procedure well with no complications.

„.iud-insertion*

58300

„.iud-removal*

58301

„.iud-removal-proc

Intrauterine Device (IUD) Removal

After appropriate discussion of risks and benefits of IUD removal, informed consent was obtained. The patient was placed in the dorsal lithotomy position, and a speculum was inserted. The IUD strings were seen at external os and grasped with sterile ring forceps and removed without difficulty. An IUD hook or other device was not needed. Patient tolerated the procedure well without complications.

Back up contraception was discussed.

,.iud-surveillance#

IUD surveillance
IUD strings visualized.
No complications.
Reassured some spotting expected during the first few months.
Counseled on safe sex to avoid STDs.
F/u prn.

,.menopause

Menopause
Onset: less than 10 years.
Patient c/o hot flashes and night sweats.
Interfering with daily activities, bothersome.
Patient tried behavioral/lifestyle modifications for at least 3 months without adequate response.

,.menopause#

Menopause / hot flashes
Trial of non-hormonal therapies.
Black cohosh/soy isoflavones.
Consider paroxetine or venlafaxine.

,.menopause#HRT

Menopause / hot flashes
Failed non-hormonal therapies.
Starting HRT. Trial for 6 months. No longer than 10 years.
Discussed benefits and risks. Pt demonstrate understanding.
No contraindications. Low CVD risk score.

,.menopause-HRT

Menopause
Onset: less than 10 years.
Patient c/o hot flashes and night sweats.
Interfering with daily activities, bothersome.
Patient tried behavioral/lifestyle modifications for at least 3 months without adequate response.
Patient is interested in HRT.
Denies any vaginal bleeding.
No h/o liver disease, VTE, breast or endometrial cancer, CAD, CVA.
No first-degree family hx of breast cancer.
No hypertriglyceridemia.
No history of hysterectomy.
Patient does not smoke.
Not treated for HTN or DM.

,.nexplanon-proc

Nexplanon insertion

Discussed contraceptive means available including IUD, nuvaring, combination oral contraceptives, and Nexplanon.
She wishes to proceed with Nexplanon.
Urine HCG obtained and is ***NEGATIVE***
Benefits and risks discussed with the patient.
Site: _left arm
Sterile preparation with Betadine.
Insertion site was selected 10 cm from medial epicondyle and marked along with guiding site using sterile marker.
Procedure area was prepped and draped in a sterile fashion. 5 mL of 2% lidocaine without epinephrine used for subcutaneous anesthesia. Anesthesia confirmed.
Nexplanon trocar was inserted subcutaneously and then Nexplanon capsule delivered subcutaneously.

Trocar was removed from the insertion site.
Nexplanon capsule was palpated by provider and patient to assure satisfactory placement.
Estimated blood loss: minimal.
Dressings applied: Adhesive Dressing.
Followup: The patient tolerated the procedure well without complications. Standard post-procedure care is explained and return precautions are given.

,.nexplanon*J

J7307

,.nexplanon-insertion*

11981

,.nexplanon-removal-reins*

11983

,.nexplanon-removal*

11982

,.nst/afi

\# NST/AFI
TOCO: none.
NST: baseline 150, mod variability, accels, no decels . cat I.
AFI 9.56
NST/AFI f/u.

,.pcos

PCOS
Pt is obese.
No hirsutism.
Irregular menstrual periods.
+ infertility.

,.pcos#

PCOS
With infertility and desiring fertility.
Weight loss.
Trial of metformin.

,.pelvic-organ-prolapse

Pt c/o sensation of vaginal pressure.
Denies any vaginal protrusion/bulge.
H/o vaginal deliveries.
Denies urinary incontinence.
reports urinary retention.
+ pelvic pain.
C/o sexual dysfunction/dyspareunia.

,.pelvic-organ-prolapse#

Pelvic organ prolapse
Symptomatic.
Discussed conservative tx w/ vaginal pessaries.
As well as surgical repair options.

,.pid#

PID
Ceftriaxone 250 IM given.
Rx doxycycline 100 mg po bid x 14 days.
Sent GC/CT.
Return if symptoms fail to improve or worsen.

,.plan-b

Pt requesting emergency contraception.
She had unprotected vaginal intercourse and wishes to reduce her risk of pregnancy.
Intercourse <5 days ago.
Requesting oral med (plan B).
LMP: wks ago.

,.plan-b#

Emergency contraception.
<120 hrs after unprotected intercourse.
Start medication ASAP.
Rx for Levonorgestrel (Plan B).
Repeat dosing of EC if vomiting med within 3 hrs of ingestion.
Perform pregnancy test if menses delayed more than 1 wk.

,.pms-hpi

PMS
Pt c/o depressed mood, irritability, and internal tension just before menses.
+ labile mood.
+ headaches.
+ breast tenderness, bloating.

,.pms#

Premenstrual Syndrome
Mixed somatic and behavioral symptoms.
Trial of oral contraceptives.
Lifestyle modification. Exercise, relaxation, and CBT.
Consider SSRI if not improving.

,.postpartum

The patient had a vaginal delivery on _ and is _ weeks postpartum.
Type of laceration or episiotomy: _
Lochia: +
Difficulty with urination: no.
Difficulty with hemorrhoids: no.
No difficulties breastfeeding.
Denies feeling depressed or difficulties handling the baby.
Desires contraception.

,.postpartum#

Postpartum
D/c prenatal vitamins.
Discussed symptoms of postpartum depression.
Contraception: _
Follow up prn.

,.pregnancy

Here for pregnancy test.
LMP: 1/10/16
 ICON +
Planned pregnancy, was not using any contraceptive.
Pt is G1P1
Had a NSVD 4 yrs ago, no perinatal complications.

No fam hx of congenital problems.
Wishes to establish prenatal care here.
Pt does not smoking, drinking, or using any drugs.
Lives at home w/ husband and daughter.
Feels safe at home.

,.pregnancy#

Pregnancy
G2P1 @ 6W1D.
EDD 10/16/16 by LMP.
Counseled on nutrition and wt gain.
Rx prenatal MV.
Sent for OB panel, HIV, and U.Cx
Vaginal bleeding, and spontaneous abortion signs and symptoms reviewed, if present go to hospital
OB intake done by nurse.
Nurse will call back for initial OB visit appt.

,.prenatal

Here for prenatal care.
No VB or UC.
+ FM.
+ FHT.
See ACOG.

,.prenatal#1

Prenatal care
G1P0 w/ IUP @ 13 wks 3 d.
Counseled on nutrition and wt gain.
OB panel utd.
MSAFP#1 done (10-13).
Nuchal US done (10-13).

Vaginal bleeding, and spontaneous abortion signs and symptoms reviewed, if present go to hospital.
f/u in 4 wks.

,.prenatal#2

Prenatal care
G1P0 w/ IUP @ 28 wks 3 d.
Counseled on nutrition and wt gain.
Vaginal bleeding, and spontaneous abortion signs and symptoms reviewed, if present go to hospital.
US anatomy screen done.
MSAFP #2 done (16-20).
F/u in 4 wks.

,.prenatal#2.1

Prenatal care
G1P0 w/ IUP @ 34 wks 3 d.
Counseled on nutrition and wt gain.
Preterm labor signs and symptoms reviewed, if present go to hospital.
FM/kick counting if decreased fetal movement.
Breastfeeding class.
Hospital registration (32).
F/u in 2 wks.

,.prenatal#3

Prenatal care
G1P0 w/ IUP @ 36 wks 3 d.
Counseled on nutrition and wt gain.
Preterm labor signs and symptoms reviewed, if present go to hospital.
FM/kick counting if decreased fetal movement.
GBS done (35-37).
Hospital registration (32).

Carseat.
F/u in 2 wks.

,.vaginal-atrophy

Vaginal atrophy
C/o painful intercourse, dryness, itchiness.
No vaginal bleeding.

,.vaginal-atrophy#

Vaginal atrophy
Trial of vaginal moisturizers and lubricants.
(Replents, KY-Jelly).
Avoid long term use of Premarin.

,.vaginitis

C/o vaginal discharge for the past days.
Endorses vaginal odor.
Denies vaginal itching/burning/irritation.
Denies dysuria, frequency, urgency or hematuria.
Denies abdominal/pelvic pain.
No recent use of abx.
OTC tx: none.
Sexually active. no new partners.
LMP: wks ago.

,.vaginitis#BV

Vaginitis
Likely Bacterial Vaginosis. Nitrazine pH >4.5, wet mount: clue cells. thin, white d/c. +whiff test.
  Tx w/ metronidazole 500 PO bid x 7 days. avoid alcohol during tx.

Return if symptoms not improving.

,.vaginitis#candida

Vaginitis
Likely Candida Vaginitis. Nitrazine pH <4.5, KOH: pseudohyphae. white, cottage-cheese-like d/c.
  Tx w/ Clotrimazole 2% vag crm x3 days/ Fluconazole 150 mg PO x1.
Return if symptoms not improving.

,.vaginitis#trichomona

Vaginitis
Likely Trichomoniasis. Nitrazine pH >7. micro: trichomonads. copious malodorous, yellow-green d/c w/ vulvar irritation, strawberry cervix. fishy odor.
  Tx w/ metronidazole 2g PO x1. avoid alcohol during tx. rx tx for sex partner. no intercourse until partner tx.
Return if symptoms not improving.

,.vaginitis-PE

General: NAD.
Abdomen: soft, non tender.
Vagina: Healthy pink mucosa, _ discharge, no lesions.
Cervix: No lesions, no cervical motion tenderness, _ discharge.
Ext genitalia: Normal, no lesions.
Inguinal lymph nodes not enlarged.

11 MUSCULOSKELETAL (ORTHO/SPORTS/PODIATRY)

,.ac-joint-inj*

20600

,.ac-joint-inj

AC joint injection, Right
AC joint was marked and then prepped in the usual sterile fashion. Using a 25 gauge 1.5 inch needle, 1 mL of lidocaine and triamcinolone - 10 mg was injected into the joint space without difficulty. After injection, the joint was passively moved through the full range of motion and a sterile dressing was applied. The patient tolerated the procedure well. Aftercare discussed.

,.achilles-tendinitis

Pt c/o a sensation of fullness/nodule in the back of the leg/posterior ankle.
C/o localized pain during and following activity.

,.achilles-tendinitis#

Achilles tendinosis
Activity modification.
Ice when symptomatic.
Prn NSAIDs.
Achilles tendon taping with ankle strapping for support done in clinic.

,.achilles-tendinitis-PE

Right achilles tendon with localized tenderness proximal to its insertion. Increased thickness and tender nodule palpated. Negative Thompson test.

,.ankle-PE

Ankle Exam:
Right ankle examined.
No edema.
No TTP over the posterior or tip of medial/lateral malleoli, proximal 5th MT, or Navicular.
Neg squeeze test.
Full ROM.
Full overall Strength.
ATFL Intact on Anterior Drawer.
Deltoid Ligament Intact.

,.ankle-pain

Pt c/o ankle pain, right.
Location: lateral.
Worsens with ambulation.
No symptoms of instability.
No injury.
No h/o surgery.

‚..ankle-pain-acute

Pt c/o ankle pain, right.
Sustained injury days ago.
Felt immediate pain on the lateral side.
Was able to ambulate after incident.
Denies h/o previous ankle injuries.
Has used NSAIDs with minor relief.

‚..ankle-sprain#

Ankle sprain, right
Continue conservative management.
Weight-bearing.
Pain control.
ROM and strength exercises.
Ankle brace.

‚..ankle-sprain#acute

Ankle sprain, right
Followed Ottawa rules and pt was sent for x-ray.
X-ray was unremarkable, with no fracture.
Limited wt bearing.
Early mobilization.
Range-of-motion exercises.
Ice.
Ankle brace.
Elevation.
Pain control.
RTC if condition worsening or not improving in a week.

‚..back-PE-low

Lower back: no obvious deformities.

Right paraspinal area tender to palpation. Full ROM.

,.back-PE-upp

Upper back: no obvious deformities.
Right trap area tender to palpation. Neck full ROM.

,.back-pain-low

C/o lower back pain x days.
No radiation.
Pain described as sharp.
Exacerbated by bending.
Relieved by rest.
No assoc sx like: fever, bowel/bladder incontinence, and neurologic deficits, saddle anesthesia.
No history of steroid use, malignancy, infection, depression.
Denies any recent trauma or occupational injury.

,.back-pain-upp

C/o neck pain x days.
No radiation.
Pain described as sharp.
Exacerbated by neck rotation.
Relieved by rest.
No assoc sx like: weakness, decreased sensation, dropping objects.
No history of steroid use, malignancy, infection, depression.
Denies any recent trauma or occupational injury.

,.back-pain#acute

Lower back pain
Acute.

W/o radiculopathy.
No red flags.
Tylenol or NSAIDS as first line tx.
Rx topicals: capsaicin, lidocaine.
Physical activity as tolerated. encouraged pt to stay active.
Reassured pain will most likely resolve in a few weeks.
Consider physical therapy.
Lifestyle modification: good lifting techniques.
Printed back exercises handout.
 Short term use of muscle relaxant.
 Discouraged long-term use of opioids.

,.back-pain#chronic

Lower back pain
Chronic (>12 wks).
W/o radiculopathy.
No red flags.
Tylenol or NSAIDS as first line tx.
Rx topicals: capsaicin, lidocaine.
Behavioral modification: wt loss.
Printed back exercises handout.
Consider Cymbalta.
Consider cognitive behavioral therapy.
Consider referral for pain management.
 Discouraged long-term use of opioids.
 Consider epidural steroid injection for chronic radicular pain from disk herniation.

,.back-pain#upp

Upper back pain
W/o radiculopathy.
No red flags.
Tylenol or NSAIDS as first line tx.
Rx topicals: capsaicin, lidocaine.

Consider physical therapy.
Printed back exercises handout.

,.back-pain-PE

Rising from chair: normal.
Ambulation: normal.
Flexibility of spine: normal.
Toe/heel walk: normal.
No midline spine tenderness.
Tender to palpation on _right paraspinal area.
ROM: full extension of the leg at the knee.
Full dorsiflexion of the great toe.
Full plantar flexion of toe and foot.
Sensation on lower extremities: normal.
Strength on lower extremities: 5/5.
Pedal pulses: present.
DTR. patellar 2+, ankle reflex 2+.
Negative straight leg raise test.

,.bicep-tendinitis

Pt c/o anterior shoulder pain, right.
Exacerbated by lifting or pulling.
No h/o injury.

,.bicep-tendinitis#

Bicep-tendinitis, right
Rest, ice, NSAIDs.
PT.
Consider steroid injection if not improving.

,.bicep-tendinitis-PE

Right shoulder: tenderness over the bicipital groove. Pain reproduced with flexion of the arm against resistance.
+ Speed test.
+ Yergason test.

,.bicep-tendinitis-inj

Biceps tendon injection, Right
Bicipital tendon (long head) area of maximal tenderness was marked and then prepped in the usual sterile fashion. Using a 25 gauge 1.5 inch needle, 1 mL of lidocaine and triamcinolone - 20 mg was injected without difficulty. After injection, the patient was able to move the biceps through the full range of motion and a sterile dressing was applied. The patient tolerated the procedure well. Aftercare discussed.

,.biceps-tend-inj*

20550

,.buddy-tape

Right middle finger buddy taped to index finger.

,.buddy-tape*toes

29550

,.buddy-tape*fingers

29280

,.callus

Pt c/o foot callus, right.
Causing considerable amount of pain and discomfort.

,.callus#

Callus
Callus debulked by pairing skin w/ blade.
Apply salicylic acid plaster patch and replace qhs.
RTC if lesion does not resolve in 1-2 wks.

,.callus-PE

Right foot:
diffuse skin thickening on
 plantar aspect of prominent metatarsal
 dorsal aspect of toe joint

,.callus-paring-1*

11055

,.callus-paring-2-4*

11056

,.callus-paring-proc

Pairing of callus
Location: _
Using a no. 15 scalpel blade the hyperkeratotic tissue from _callus was removed by gradually shaving the lesion.

Patient tolerated procedure well.

,.carpal-tunnel

C/o numbness of hands.
Nighttime worsening.
Numbness in the median nerve distribution.
Symptoms are intermittent.
Onset is gradual.
Denies weakness of hand.
Hand intensive labor at work.

,.carpal-tunnel#

Carpal tunnel
Wrist splint.
NSAIDs.
Consider steroid injection if no improvement.

,.carpal-tunnel*

20526

,.carpal-tunnel-PE

Normal motor exam - no wasting of thenar eminence, normal pincer grasp.
Normal sensation.
+ tinel sign.
+ phalen sign.
+ compression test.

,.carpal-tunnel-inj

Carpal tunnel injection, right
Informed consent was obtained from the patient. The volar aspect of the wrist was prepared with alcohol x3 and rested at a 30 degree angle on a rolled-up towel. The palmaris longus tendon was identified and a 25 gauge 1" needle was used to enter the carpal tunnel at the distal wrist crease and ulnar to the palmaris longus tendon. The needle was advanced through the carpal tunnel without any difficulty. No paresthesias were elicited. A mixture of 1 mL of lidocaine 1% w/o epi and 1 mL of 40 mg triamcinolone was injected . The medications flowed freely without any difficulty. After the procedure, the patient clenched and unclenched the fingers of both hands for a period of two minutes to distribute the medication. There were no complications throughout the procedure and good relief of symptoms following the procedure.

POST PROCEDURE INSTRUCTIONS: The patient has been asked to report to us any redness, swelling, inflammation, or fevers. The patient has been asked to restrict the use of the extremity for the next 24 hours.

,.coccydynia

Pt c/o coccyx pain.
Pain occurs while sitting or transitioning between standing and sitting.
Described as ache.
Radiates to lumbar spine and thigh.
Denies any injuries.

,.coccydynia#

\# Coccydynia
Recommended rest.
Adjustment in seating with U-shaped/wedge shape cushions to relieve pressure on the coccyx.
Pain control with analgesics/ sitz baths.

,.coccydynia-PE

Tenderness on palpation and movement of the tip of the coccyx.

,.corn#

Corn
Corn debulked by pairing skin w/ blade.
Apply salicylic acid plaster patch and replace qhs.
Short soaks and pumice stone debridement at home.
Footwear with extra toe space.
RTC if lesion does not resolve in 1-2 wks.

,.corn-PE

Right foot: plantar aspect / toe cleft.
Diffuse thickening with central "core" that is hyperkeratotic and tender to palpation.

,.corn-paring-1*

11055

,.corn-paring-2-4*

11056

,.corn-paring-procedure

Pairing of corn
Location: _right foot.
Using a no. 15 scalpel blade the hyperkeratotic tissue from corn was removed by gradually shaving the lesion.

Patient tolerated procedure well.

,.cyst-mucous

Patient has a history of right index finger DIP joint osteoarthritis.
Status post joint injection.
Patient complains of a cyst that is enlarging on the site of injection.

,.cyst-mucous#

Digital mucous cyst
Aspirated.
Wound care.

,.cyst-mucous-PE

Right index finger DIP joint: digital mucous cyst on radial aspect.

,.cyst-mucous-asp

Digital mucous cyst aspiration
Right index finger
Area was prepped in the usual sterile fashion.
Ethyl chloride was used for topical anesthesia.
An 18 G needle tip was inserted in the center of the cyst.
Cyst contents were manually extruded.
Pt tolerated procedure well.
Sterile bandaid applied.

,.cyst-mucous-asp*

26160

,.dequervain

Pt complains of pain in the base of the _right thumb for months. Worsening when lifting heavy objects.

,.dequervain#

\# De Quervain tenosynovitis, right
NSAIDs and splinting.
Consider first dorsal compartment steroid injection.

,.dequervain-PE

Right wrist: no obvious deformity, no edema, full ROM, radial styloid area w/ mild tenderness to palpation. + finkelstein test.

,.dequervain-inj

De Quervain tenosynovitis injection, Right
Explained nature of condition to pt.
Refractory to medical management.
Pt opted for steroid tendon injection.
Steroid injection (10 mg triamcinolone + 0.5 mL plain lidocaine) between abductor pollicis longus and Extensor pollicis brevis tendon was given.
Aftercare and return precautions discussed w/ pt.
Continue NSAIDs/Tylenol PRN.
Thumb spica wrist brace given to patient.

,.dequervain-inj*

20550

,.dry-needling-proc

Dry needling/trigger point injection
Discussed treatment options, risks, benefits and alternatives. Patient opted for trigger point injection.
Trigger point injection/dry needling to left lateral epicondyle was given.
Patient signed informed consent. A 35 G needle was used.
Procedure was well tolerated.
Aftercare and return precautions discussed with patient.

,.epicondylitis

Patient c/o elbow pain.
During or following flexion and extension.
Exacerbates with repetitive movement or occupational activity.
Denies decreased grip strength.
Located on lateral aspect of _ elbow.

,.epicondylitis#

Epicondylitis
Rest + ice + NSAIDs + brace/strap.
PT exercises.
If no improvement consider steroid injection.

,.epicondylitis*

20551

,.epicondylitis-lat-PE

Tenderness on lateral epicondyle. Pain during resisted wrist extension/ext rotation.

,.epicondylitis-lat-inj

Lateral epicondylitis steroid injection, Right
After discussion of risks and benefits of steroid injection, including but not limited to infection, bleeding, discomfort with injection, adverse reaction to protein, and possibility of no improvement in pain symptoms patient gave verbal and written consent. Time-out performed and site of injection was verified and patient identified by name and DOB.
Elbow was prepped with isopropyl alcohol x 3. Ethyl chloride used for local anesthesia. 40 mg of kenalog mixed with 3 cc of 1%lidocaine w/o epi was then injected into lateral epicondyle using a 25 gauge needle using the fanning approach. Patient tolerated procedure well and was hemostatic at conclusion. Aftercare instructions provided, including returning to clinic if knees become warm, red, or more painful in the next 72 hours and limiting activity for the next 24-48 hours.

,.epicondylitis-med-PE

Tenderness on the medial epicondyle. Pain during resisted wrist/forearm pronation/flexion.

,.epicondylitis-med-inj

Medial epicondylitis steroid injection, Right
After discussion of risks and benefits of steroid injection, including but not limited to infection, bleeding, discomfort with injection, adverse reaction to protein, and possibility of no improvement in pain symptoms patient gave verbal and written consent. Time-out performed and site of injection was verified and patient identified by name and DOB.

Elbow was prepped with isopropyl alcohol x 3. Ethyl chloride used for local anesthesia. 40 mg of kenalog mixed with 3 cc of 1%lidocaine w/o epi was then injected into medial epicondyle using a 25 gauge needle using the fanning approach. Patient tolerated procedure well and was hemostatic at conclusion. Aftercare instructions provided, including returning to clinic if knees become warm, red, or more painful in the next 72 hours and limiting activity for the next 24-48 hours.

,.fibromyalgia

Fibromyalgia
Compliant with amitriptyline.
Using tylenol/NSAIDs prn pain.
No recent exacerbations.
Good adherence to exercise and behavioral therapy.
No sleep disruption.
Not interfering with daily functioning.

,.fibromyalgia#

Fibromyalgia
Stable.
Continue amitriptyline, same dose.
Continue analgesics prn pain.
Non-pharmacologic therapies:
Encouraged pt to exercise early during the day.
Advised on sleep hygiene.
Advised on pt support including National Fibromyalgia Assoc. fmaware.org
Consider cognitive behavioral therapy.

,.foosh

Pt c/o wrist pain, left.
After falling on an out-stretched hand with the wrist in extension.
No deformities noted.

Reports swelling after injury.
Denies any previous wrist injuries or surgery.

,.foosh-PE

Left wrist
No obvious deformities such as "dinner-fork".
Some edema and area tender to palpation.
Anatomic snuffbox not tender to palpation.
Limited ROM d/t pain.
NVI.
Elbow and shoulder joints wnl.

,.foot-pain-metatarsal

Pt c/o foot pain, right
Causing pain around the ball of the foot
Feels like a stone in the shoe
Worse when walking barefoot

,.foot-pain-metatarsal#

Metatarsalgia
Conservative management.
Analgesics prn.
Metatarsal pads.

,.foot-pain-PE

Hammer toes.
Splayed toes.
Interphalangeal toes flexion contractures.
Calluses on the dorsum of proximal interphalangeal joints.
Calluses over the plantar metatarsophalangeal joints.

,.ganglion-cyst

Pt c/o mass on wrist.
Reports some pain.
Increases in size after activity.
Denies any numbness of fingers.

,.ganglion-cyst#

Ganglion cyst
W/o neurovascular compromise.
Activity modification and analgesia.
Cyst aspiration discussed.
Splint recommended.

,.ganglion-cyst*

20612

,.ganglion-cyst-PE

1x1 cm transilluminating subcutaneous mass on wrist. Not tender to palpation. Soft.

,.ganglion-cyst-proc

Ganglion cyst aspiration
Wrist, right
After discussion of the risks, benefits and alternative therapies available, the patient elected to proceed. After obtaining informed consent, the patient's identity, procedure, and site were verified during a pause prior to proceeding

with the minor surgical procedure as per universal protocol recommendations.
Area was cleansed with povidone/iodine swabs. Ethyl chloride was sprayed in the area for anesthesia. An 18-gauge needle attached to a 5 cc syringe was then used to aspirate the ganglion cyst. 1cc mixture of 1% plain lidocaine and 20 mg of triamcinolone where then injected. Hemostasis was obtained by pressure. There were no complications.

,.gout

Gout
Patient has had no attacks during last year.
Does not complain of joint pain.
Has not noticed any tofi formation.
Compliant with uric acid-lowering agent. Allopurinol.
Not using NSAIDs, colchicine, or steroid.
Not using diuretics.
Patient is not drinking alcohol/beer. Reduced intake of meats/seafood and dairy products.

,.gout#

Gout
Controlled.
Continue with uric acid-lowering agent. No changes in management.
Uric acid check (q6mo, goal <6).
CMP, CBC check (q6mo).
Recommended wt loss. Avoid food with high purine content.

,.gout-flare

Gout
Patient complains of joint pain.
Right toe Drinks alcohol. High intake of meats/seafood and dairy products.

Using NSAIDs with mild relief of pain.
Not using diuretics.

,.gout-flare#

Gout, acute
Short course of high dose NSAIDs.
Consider steroid injection.
Check uric acid to confirm dx of gout.
Consider starting allopurinol if high, 2 wks after acute episode.

,.hallux-valgus

Hallux valgus
C/o painful bilateral big toe.
Exacerbated when using closed shoes.
Present for years.
Worsening.

,.hallux-valgus#

Hallux valgus, bilateral
Footwear adaptation to relieve pressure.
Consider surgical repair if significant deformity causing pain and affecting daily life.

,.hallux-valgus-PE

Lateral deviation of the hallux on the first metatarsal, some erythema on the medial bursa protecting the joint.

,.hamstring-sprain

Pt c/o pain in the posterior thigh, left. x1 mo.
Gradual onset.
Sudden onset after running jumping.
Pt felt a tearing sensation.

,.hamstring-sprain#

Hamstring sprain, left
Home physical therapy exercises.
Active ROM/strengthening. Isometric exercises.
TENS. Ice.
Pain control.
Gradual return to play. Importance of warm-up/stretching.
Risk of reinjury.

,.hamstring-sprain-PE

Left hamstring area: no masses, tender to palpation, pain reproduced with resisted flexion. Knee with full ROM.

,.hip-PE

Hip Exam: Right
Soft tissue swelling not appreciated.
Gait: antalgic.
Trochanteric not TTP.
Sciatic Notch not TTP.
Anterior hip TTP.
Full overall ROM and Strength.
Ober's Test: neg.
Log Roll: +
FADERs: +
FABIRs: +

NVI.

,.hip-oa

Pt c/o hip pan, right.
Denies any injuries.
No Locking/Catching.
No Snapping.
Worsens with ambulation.
Alleviating Factors: NSAIDs.
No Prior Injuries/Surgeries.

,.hip-oa#

Hip OA, right
NSAIDs/tylenol prn.
ROM and strengthening exercises.
Discussed wt loss.
Consider intra-articular corticosteroid injection.

,.ingrown-toenail

Patient c/o pain, redness, and swelling of corner of toenail.
Affecting right big toe.
No purulence.
Reports no previous episode.
No h/o trauma.
Proper fitting shoes.

,.ingrown-toenail#

Ingrown toenail, right
Well-fitted shoes with a wide toe box recommended.

Trim toenails properly. Avoid cutting back to the lateral margins in a curved pattern.
Soak toe in warm water, followed by application of topical antibiotics.

,.ingrown-toenail*

11750

,.ingrown-toenail-PE

Left big toe: medial ingrown toenail, there is edema and mild erythema of the nail fold. No purulence or ulceration.

,.ingrown-toenail-proc

Right lateral great toe partial nail avulsion:
Skin cleaned with 70% alcohol swab.
Digital block performed with 1:1 ratio of 1% Lidocaine (without Epinephrine) + 0.25% Bupivacaine.
Area was prepped in usual sterile fashion with 10% Iodine swab and sterile drapes, and sterile gloves used.
Nail elevator used to separate lateral aspect of nail from the nail bed.
Hemostat used to clamp lateral aspect of nail.
Podiatry scissors used to cut lateral 1/4 of the nail.
Nail removed by turning hemostat clockwise and the nail was pulled out easily.
Nailbed cauterized with silver nitrate also to achieve hemostasis. in addition to applying direct pressure.
Neosporin applied and toe was wrapped with gauze and kerlix bandage roll.

,.injection#

Explained nature of condition to pt.
Refractory to medical management.

Pt opted for steroid intra-articular injection.
Steroid injection to _ was given.
Aftercare and return precautions discussed w/ pt.
Continue NSAIDs/Tylenol PRN.
Gave handout with information about condition and stretch/strengthening exercises.
F/u PRN.

,.injection*intermediate-joint (TMJ,AC,W,E,A)

20605

,.injection*major-joint

20610

,.injection*small-joint

20600

,.injection-knee

Knee steroid injection, right
After discussion of risks and benefits of steroid injection, including but not limited to infection, bleeding, discomfort with injection, adverse reaction to protein, and possibility of no improvement in pain symptoms patient gave verbal and written consent. Time-out performed and site of injection was verified and patient identified by name and DOB. Knee was prepped with betadine x 3. Ethyl chloride used for local anesthesia. 40 mg of triamcinolone mixed with 4 cc of 1%lidocaine w/o epi was then injected into knee using a 22 gauge needle using the inferolateral approach. Patient tolerated procedure well and was hemostatic at conclusion. Aftercare instructions provided, including returning to clinic if knees become warm,

red, or more painful in the next 72 hours and limiting activity for the next 24-48 hours.

,.injection-shoulder

Right shoulder injection
After discussion of risks and benefits of corticosteroid injection, including but not limited to infection, bleeding, discomfort with injection, skin atrophy or color changes, injury to surrounding structures, elevated blood sugar, and the possibility of no improvement in pain symptoms patient gave verbal and written consent.
Time-out performed and site of injection was verified and patient identified by name and DOB.
Shoulder was prepped with betadine x 3. Ethyl chloride used for local anesthesia.
4 cc of 1% lidocaine and 40 mg of triamcinolone was mixed and then injected into the glenohumeral joint using a posterior approach with a 22 gauge needle.
Patient tolerated procedure well and was hemostatic at conclusion.
Aftercare instructions provided, including returning to clinic if shoulder becomes warm, red, or more painful in the next 72 hours and limiting activity for the next 24-48 hours.

,.itbandSd

Pt c/o sharp and burning pain superior to right lateral knee.
Radiates proximally to lateral thigh.
Denies injuries. Exercises frequently.
Workout includes biking and machine weights for legs.
Worse at night after activities.
Similar episode a couple of years ago.

,.itbandSd#

IT band Sd, right

NSAIDs for pain and inflammation.
Activity modification.

,.itbandSd-PE

+ Noble test, w/ compression tenderness 2cm proximal to the lateral femoral epicondyle on extension.
+ Ober test, showing tightness of the IT band.

,.knee#

Knee PFPS, right
NSAIDs/tylenol prn.
Local analgesia with capsaicin topical.
Quadriceps-strengthening exercises.
Knee brace.
Discussed wt loss.
Consider intra-articular corticosteroid injection.

,.knee-PE

Right Knee
No effusion.
Normal gait.
+ crepitus.
Not TTP.
Full ROM and overall strength.
Normal patellar glide laxity.
Neg apprehension test.
Intact ligaments w/ valgus and varus stress; anterior and posterior drawer.
Instability on single leg squad.

,.knee-asp/inj

Knee aspiration & injection, right

After discussion of risks and benefits of aspiration and steroid injection, including but not limited to infection, bleeding, discomfort with injection, adverse reaction to protein and possibility of no improvement in pain symptoms patient gave verbal and written consent. Time-out performed and site of aspiration was verified and patient identified by name and DOB. Knee was prepped with betadine x 3. Ethyl chloride used for local anesthesia. 5 mL of lidocaine 1% with epinephrine were injected subcutaneously and into soft tissues. using a 25 gauge needle. Then using an 18 gauge needle using the inferolateral approach _60 mL of yellow cloudy fluid were aspirated. Subsequently 40 mg of triamcinolone mixed with 4 cc of 1%lidocaine w/o epi was then injected. Patient tolerated procedure well and was hemostatic at conclusion. Aftercare instructions provided, including returning to clinic if knees become warm, red, or more painful in the next 72 hours and limiting activity for the next 24-48 hours.

,.knee-aspiration

Knee aspiration, right
After discussion of risks and benefits of aspiration, including but not limited to infection, bleeding, discomfort with injection, and the possibility of no improvement in pain symptoms patient gave verbal and written consent. Time-out performed and site of aspiration was verified and patient identified by name and DOB. Knee was prepped with betadine x 3. Ethyl chloride used for local anesthesia. 5 mL of lidocaine 1% with epinephrine were injected subcutaneously and into soft tissues. using a 25 gauge needle. Then using an 18 gauge needle using the inferolateral approach _60 mL of yellow cloudy fluid were aspirated. Patient tolerated procedure well and was hemostatic at conclusion. Aftercare instructions provided, including returning to clinic if knees become warm, red, or more painful in the next 72 hours and limiting activity for the next 24-48 hours.

,.knee-inj

Knee steroid injection, right
After discussion of risks and benefits of steroid injection, including but not limited to infection, bleeding, discomfort with injection, adverse reaction to

protein, and possibility of no improvement in pain symptoms patient gave verbal and written consent. Time-out performed and site of injection was verified and patient identified by name and DOB. Knee was prepped with betadine x 3. Ethyl chloride used for local anesthesia. 40 mg of triamcinolone mixed with 4 cc of 1%lidocaine w/o epi was then injected into knee using a 22 gauge needle using the inferolateral approach. Patient tolerated procedure well and was hemostatic at conclusion. Aftercare instructions provided, including returning to clinic if knees become warm, red, or more painful in the next 72 hours and limiting activity for the next 24-48 hours.

,.knee-inj*

20610

,.knee-inj-viscosuppl

Knee viscosupplementation injection, right
After discussion of risks and benefits of hyaluronic acid injection, including but not limited to infection, bleeding, discomfort with injection, adverse reaction to protein, and possibility of no improvement in pain symptoms patient gave verbal and written consent. Time-out performed and site of injection was verified and patient identified by name and DOB. Right knee was prepped with betadine x 3. Ethyl chloride used for local anesthesia. 2.5 mL of hyaluronic acid _(Supartz) were then injected into knee using a 22 gauge needle using the inferolateral approach. Patient tolerated procedure well and was hemostatic at conclusion. Aftercare instructions provided, including returning to clinic if knees become warm, red, or more painful in the next 72 hours and limiting activity for the next 24-48 hours.

,.knee-meniscus

Pt c/o knee pain, right.
Hx of knee trauma.
Knee swelling after trauma.

Sensation of instability, buckling/catching.

,.knee-patellar-tendonitis

Pt c/o right knee pain, swelling and stiffness for a few weeks.
Localized to anterior aspect.
Pt plays sports, frequent jumping.
No h/o previous injury.

,.knee-patellofem sd

Pt c/o knee pain, Right.
Insidious onset.
Ill-defined ache localized to the anterior knee.
Aggravated by climbing stairs., walking after prolonged sitting.

,.knee-OA

Knee osteoarthritis
Pt c/o pain w/ activity & relieved by rest.
Pain well controlled with NSAIDs.

,.knee-OA#

Right knee osteoarthritis
NSAIDs/tylenol prn.
Local analgesia with capsaicin topical.
Quadriceps-strengthening exercises.
Knee brace.
Discussed wt loss.
Consider intra-articular corticosteroid injection.

,.morton-neuroma

Patient complains of pain and numbness of left foot and toes. Interdigital 3/4th digits.
Pain that increases with activity and is usually felt on the plantar surface between the third and fourth toes.
Pt also c/o paraesthesias in the same area at night.

,.morton-neuroma#

Morton neuroma
Conservative management.
Wide toe-box shoes and Metatarsal pad recommended.

,.morton-neuroma-PE

Positive Mulder sign on 3-4 toe web space.

,.neck-pain

Pt c/o neck pain x days.
No radiation.
Pain described as sharp.
Exacerbated by neck rotation.
Relieved by rest.
No assoc sx like: weakness, decreased sensation, dropping objects.
No history of steroid use, malignancy, infection, depression.
Denies any recent trauma or occupational injury.

,.neck-pain#

Neck/upper back pain
W/o radiculopathy.
No red flags.

Tylenol or NSAIDS as first line tx.
Rx topicals: capsaicin, lidocaine.
Consider physical therapy.
Printed exercises handout.

,.neck-pain-PE

Bilateral upper back /neck tender to palpation on trapezius muscle area.
Negative Spurling's test.

,.olecranon-bursitis

Pt c/o pain and swelling on right elbow, at site of bursa.
Denies any recent trauma.
Denies any fevers or chills.

,.olecranon-bursitis#

Olecranon bursitis
Conservative management and analgesia.
Rest + Ice + Compression.
Consider steroid injection.

,.olecranon-bursitis-PE

Right elbow with edema and erythema at the site of bursa. Warm to touch and tender to palpation.

,.olecranon-bursitis-inj/asp

Olecranon bursitis aspiration and injection, right

Elbow was marked and then prepped in the usual sterile fashion. Using a 20 gauge 1.5 inch needle, _5 ml of serosanguineous fluid was aspirated from the joint space without difficulty. A mixture of 2 cc of 1% lidocaine and 20 mg of triamcinolone were then injected. After aspiration and injection, the joint was passively moved through the full range of motion and a sterile dressing was applied. The patient tolerated the procedure well. Aftercare discussed.

,.olecranon-bursitis-inj/asp*

20605

,.patellar-bursitis

Pt c/o anterior knee pain.
No swelling or redness.
Worsens w/ kneeling. Relief w/ rest.
Occupation requiring excessive kneeling.

,.pes-anserine*

20605

,.pes-anserine-inj

Pes anserine injection, right
After discussion of risks and benefits of steroid injection, including but not limited to infection, bleeding, discomfort with injection, adverse reaction to protein, and possibility of no improvement in pain symptoms patient gave verbal and written consent. Time-out performed and site of injection was verified and patient identified by name and DOB. Knee was prepped with isopropyl alcohol x 3. Ethyl chloride used for local anesthesia. 20 mg of kenalog mixed with 1 cc of 1%lidocaine w/o epi was then injected into pes anserine bursa/point of maximal tenderness using a 25 gauge needle.

Patient tolerated procedure well and was hemostatic at conclusion. Aftercare instructions provided, including returning to clinic if knees become warm, red, or more painful in the next 72 hours and limiting activity for the next 24-48 hours.

,.pes-planus

Flat feet, bilateral
Pt c/o pain and swelling in the medial ankle and midfoot during weight bearing.
Condition present for years.

,.pes-planus#

Pes planus, bilateral
XR ordered.
Conservative management.
NSAIDs prn.
Consider use of orthotics.
Appreciate podiatry consultation and recommendations.

,.pes-planus-PE

Bilateral visible pes planus deformity.
Inability/ pain upon attempts to perform a single-leg heel rise.
Abnormal wear of the medial heel and inner border of footwear noted.

,.piriformis-sd

Patient c/o right buttock pain that radiates to leg.
No h/o trauma or injury.
Worsens with sitting.

,.piriformis-sd#

Piriformis syndrome
Physical therapy involving strengthening of the pelvic and hip region and stretching of the piriformis. Prn analgesics.
Consider steroid injection if not improving.

,.piriformis-sd-PE

Abnormally tight and tender piriformis muscle on right buttock and positive figure-four test. Pain also reproduced with resisting external rotation.

,.piriformis-sd-inj

Injection piriformis sd, right
Piriformis muscle was located about half the distance from the sacral crest to the femoral trochanter.
Maximal point of tenderness was identified and entry point was marked.
Area was prepped in the usual sterile manner.
Injection: 40 mg of triamcinolone + 1 mL of 1% lidocaine using a 25 G 1 in needle.
The needle was inserted into the affected area and the steroid was injected.
Patient tolerated procedure well without complications.
Standard post-procedure care was explained and return precautions given.

,.piriformis-sd-inj*

20552

,.plantar-fasciitis

Patient complains of heel pain, right
Described as stabbing.

Pain exacerbated by walking barefoot.
Relieved with rest.
Pain with the first few steps after rising from a seated or lying position.
No improvement with NSAIDs.

,.plantar-fasciitis#

Plantar fasciitis
Rest.
Weight loss.
Stretching exercises.
Foot orthotics and night splint.
Consider steroid injection if not improving.

,.plantar-fasciitis*strapping

29540

,.plantar-fasciitis-PE

left foot: no tenderness to palpation on plantar medial arch, distal to insertion of calcaneus.

,.plantar-fasciitis-inj*

20550

,.plantar-fasciitis-inj

Plantar Fascia Injection, Right
Informed consent was obtained from the patient. Special mention was made of the possibility of heel pad atrophy and plantar fascia rupture. The

patient was placed in the supine position. The tender area in the medial aspect of the heel was identified by palpation. After proper preparation of the skin with antiseptic solution skin, a syringe containing 1 mL of 1% lidocaine and 40 mg of triamcinolone was attached to 1.5" 25 gauge needle. The needle was carefully advanced through the carefully identified point at a right angle to the skin, directly towards the central and medial aspect of the calcaneus. The solution was injected as a bolus at the origin of the plantar fascia. The contents of the syringe were then gently injected and flowed smoothly into the space. Subsequently the needle was removed. Pressure was applied at the site of insertion and once it was made sure there was no bleeding taking place, a small bandage was applied.

POST PROCEDURE INSTRUCTIONS: The patient has been asked to report to us any redness, swelling, inflammation, or fevers. The patient has been asked to restrict the use of the extremity for the next 24 hours.

,.ra-hands

Pt c/o bilateral hand joint pain and swelling.
Reports morning stiffness.
Fam hx of rheumatoid arthritis.

,.ra-hands#

Rheumatoid arthritis, hands
Mild to moderate ds
Treatment options discussed with the patient.
DMARDs, steroids, NSAIDs.

,.ra-hands-PE

Multiple joint deformities.
Hand w ulnar deviation and swan neck deformity of multiple fingers.

,.rice

Rest + ice + NSAIDs + brace.

,.rotator-cuff

Right shoulder pain
Patient complains of gradual onset of anterior and lateral pain.
Exacerbated by overhead activities.
Patient cannot sleep unaffected side.
Symptoms have been present for months.
Labor intensive work, carries heavy objects.
Pain relieved w/ NSAIDs.
Denies any injuries or previous surgeries.
No instability symptoms.
No numbness and tingling.

,.rotator-cuff#

Rotator cuff tendinitis
Conservative management.
ROM/strengthening exercises.
Consider steroid injection if no improvement.

,.rotator-cuff-PE

Right shoulder
No obvious deformities.
Pain with abduction past 90 degrees.
+ Hawkins.
+ Neers.
Pain w/ resisted external rotation.
Pain w/ empty-can test.
Neg scarf test.

,.rotator-cuff-inj

Shoulder injection, right
Procedure:
After discussion of risks and benefits of corticosteroid injection, including but not limited to infection, bleeding, discomfort with injection, skin atrophy or color changes, injury to surrounding structures, elevated blood sugar, and the possibility of no improvement in pain symptoms patient gave verbal and written consent.
Time-out performed and site of injection was verified and patient identified by name and DOB.
Shoulder was prepped with betadine x 3. Ethyl chloride used for local anesthesia.
4 cc of 1% lidocaine and 40 mg of triamcinolone was mixed and then injected into the glenohumeral joint using a posterior approach with a 22 gauge needle.
Patient tolerated procedure well and was hemostatic at conclusion.
Aftercare instructions provided, including returning to clinic if shoulder becomes warm, red, or more painful in the next 72 hours and limiting activity for the next 24-48 hours.

,.rotator-cuff-inj*

20610

,.shoulder

Right shoulder pain
Patient complains of gradual onset of anterior and lateral pain.
Exacerbated by overhead activities.
Patient cannot sleep unaffected side.
Symptoms have been present for months
Labor intensive work, carries heavy objects.
Pain relieved w/ NSAIDs
Denies any injuries or previous surgeries.
No instability symptoms.

No numbness and tingling.

,.shoulder-PE-labral

Labral tests
+ O'Briens, less pain with slap retention test.
+ Crank.

,.splint-finger

Static splint applied over volar aspect to immobilize right middle finger. Buddy taped to index finger.

,.splint-finger-static*

29130

,.steroid-injection*

20610

,.strapping-ankle

Right ankle strapping done in office.

,.strapping-ankle*

29540

,.strapping-knee

Right knee strapping done in office.

,.strapping-knee*

29530

,.thumb-cmc

Patient c/o right thumb pain x months .
Localized to the base of the thumb.
Aggravated by sustained grasping or pinching
or by forceful use of the thumb, such as turning a key.
Reports a sensation of thumb weakness.
Denies any injuries.

,.thumb-cmc#

\# Carpometacarpal joint osteoarthritis, right
Thumb spica splint.
NSAIDs prn.
Consider steroid injection.

,.thumb-cmc*

20600

,.thumb-cmc-PE

Right thumb: First metacarpal without any obvious deformities , full ROM.
\+ grind test.
\+ crepitus.

,.thumb-cmc-inj

Location: _right 1st CMC joint
Injection: 10 mg of triamcinolone + 0.5 mL of 2% lidocaine using a 25 G 5/8 in needle.
Entry point was marked.
Area was prepped in the usual sterile manner.
The needle was inserted into the affected area and the steroid was injected.
Patient tolerated procedure well without complications.
Standard post-procedure care was explained and return precautions given.

,.tmj-PE

Limited jaw opening, no palpable spasm of facial muscles, no facial edema. + clicking of tmj, no crepitus. No deviation of mandible.

,.tmj-inj

TMJ injection, _left
Informed consent was obtained from the patient.
With the patient's mouth in the open position the sulcus identified and marked.
The area was prepped in the usual sterile manner.
A 25 gauge needle was inserted into the affected area and a mixture of 0.5 cc of 1% lidocaine + 20 mg of triamcinolone were injected using a posterior approach at a 30-degree angle to the sagittal plane into the sulcus with the tip of the needle directed anteromedial toward the posterior aspect of the TMJ.
There were no complications during this procedure. The patient was able to move the jaw through its full range of motion.

POST PROCEDURE INSTRUCTIONS: The patient has been asked to report to us any redness, swelling, inflammation, or fevers. The patient has been asked to restrict the use of the joint for the next 24 hours.

„.tmj-inj*

20605

„.tmj-sd

TMJ sd
Pt complains of TMJ pain.
+ joint noise.
+ masticatory muscle tenderness.
Denies depression or anxiety.
C/o headaches, earaches, neck pain.

„.tmj-sd#

TMJ syndrome
Joint rest - no gum, excessive talking, soft diet.
Reduce stress.
physical therapy.
CBT/stress management.
Pain control with NSAIDs and muscle relaxants.
Consider referral to maxillofacial sx if persisting.

„.toenail-debridement

Dremel tool with sanding disc was used to debride bilateral big toenails. Patient tolerated procedure well.

„.toenail-debridement-1-5*

11720

,.toenail-debridement-6*

11721

,.toenail-trimming*

11719

,.toenail-trimming-proc

10 non-dystrophic toenails were trimmed using nail cutter.

,.triamcinolone*

J3301

,.trigger-finger

Patient complains of right 4th digit getting stuck.
Painful snapping, catching and locking during flexion.
Difficulty spontaneous extending affected digit, requiring manipulation.
Pain localized over volar aspect .
Worse in the morning.

,.trigger-finger#

Trigger-finger
Conservative management.
Corticosteroid injection recommended.

,.trigger-finger-PE

Palpable nodule in the line of the flexor digitorum superficialis, just distal to the MCP joint in the palm.

,.trigger-finger-inj

Trigger finger injection
location: _Right thumb
Tender nodule was identified in the finger's flexor tendon. Entry point was marked 1 cm distal to the nodule. Area was then prepped in the usual sterile fashion. Using a 25 gauge 5/8 inch needle, 0.5 mL of lidocaine and triamcinolone - 20 mg was injected around the nodule into the tendon sheath without difficulty. After injection, the patient was able to move finger through its full range of motion without pain. A sterile dressing was applied. The patient tolerated the procedure well. Aftercare discussed.

,.trigger-finger-inj*

20550

,.trigger-point-inj

Trigger point injection, _upper back
Discussed treatment options, risks, benefits and alternatives. Patient opted for trigger point injection. Patient signed informed consent.
Trigger point injection was given by injecting 2 cc of 0.25% marcaine on each site as below.
Patient experienced immediate relief of symptoms, >50% reduction. Procedure was well tolerated.
Aftercare and return precautions discussed with patient.
Injection sites:
trapezius, left _ / right _
splenius capitis, left _ / right _
rhomboid major, left _ / right _

latissimus dorsi, left _ / right _
gluteus maximus, left _ / right _
gluteus medius, left _ / right _

,.trigger-point-inj-steroid

Trigger point injection, _upper back
Discussed treatment options, risks, benefits and alternatives. Patient opted for trigger point injection. Patient signed informed consent.
Trigger point injection was given by injecting 2 cc of 4 mg/mL of triamcinolone mix with 0.25% marcaine on each site as below.
Patient experienced immediate relief of symptoms, >50% reduction. Procedure was well tolerated.
Aftercare and return precautions discussed with patient.
Injection sites:
trapezius, left _ / right _
splenius capitis, left _ / right _
rhomboid major, left _ / right _
latissimus dorsi, left _ / right _
gluteus maximus, left _ / right _
gluteus medius, left _ / right _

,.trigger-point-inj(1)*

20552

,.trigger-point-inj(3)*

20553

,.trochanteric-bursitis

Pt c/o pain involving the lateral aspect of the _right hip x weeks. Worsens while standing up.

,.trochanteric-bursitis#

Trochanteric bursitis, _right hip
Steroid injection given.
Conservative management.

,.trochanteric-bursitis-PE

_Right hip: tenderness to palpation at site of bursa.
Full ROM. No erythema or edema.

,.trochanteric-bursitis-inj

Trochanteric bursitis injection, right
Informed consent was obtained from the patient. With the patient lying on the examination table in the lateral decubitus position on the unaffected hip. The point of maximal tenderness on the greater trochanter was identified and marked and then prepped in the usual sterile fashion. Using a 25 gauge 1.5 inch needle, 3 mL of lidocaine and 40 mg of triamcinolone were injected into the trochanteric bursa without difficulty. After injection, the hip was passively moved through the full range of motion and a sterile dressing was applied. The patient tolerated the procedure well. Aftercare discussed.

,.trochanteric-bursitis-inj*

20610

,.ulnar-tunnel-sd

Pt complains of mild transient paresthesias mainly in the ring and small fingers.
C/o pain in the medial side of the elbow that radiates to the hand.
Denies any weakness, dropping object.
No h/o trauma or previous injury.

,.ulnar-tunnel-sd

Ulnar tunnel syndrome, right
Conservative management.
NSAIDs.
Elbow brace.
Consider referral to ortho if no improvement.

,.ulnar-tunnel-sd#

Ulnar tunnel syndrome, right
Conservative management.
NSAIDs.
Elbow brace.
Consider referral to ortho if no improvement.

,.ulnar-tunnel-sd-PE

Normal elbow ROM.
+ Tinnel sign.
+ elbow flexion test.
No masses or lesions on cubital tunnel region.
Normal overall muscle strength.
NVI.
Negative spurling's test.

,.wrist-PE

No obvious deformity. No edema. Full passive ROM of wrist on extension and flexion. Diffuse tenderness to palpation over wrist, no specific point tenderness on anatomic snuffbox. Normal sensation and motor strength.

,.wrist-inj

Right wrist injection
Area of maximal tenderness on dorsal aspect was marked and then prepped in the usual sterile fashion. Using a 25 gauge 1.5 inch needle, aspiration was attempted but no fluid was withdrawn. 0.5 mL of lidocaine and triamcinolone - 20 mg was injected without difficulty. After injection, the patient was able to move the wrist through the full range of motion and a sterile dressing was applied. The patient tolerated the procedure well. Aftercare discussed.

,.wrist-inj*

20605

12 PEDIATRICS

,.circumcision

Here w/ mother for circumcision.
Born at term.
No perinatal complications.
Normal voiding patterns.

,.circumcision#

Circumcision
Pt tolerated well the procedure.
Aftercare and return precautions discussed w/ parent.
Tylenol PRN.
Gave handout with information about procedure to parent.
Return precautions discussed w/ parent.
F/u PRN.

,.circumcision-gomco

Procedure: Infant circumcision using the Gomco clamp.

Anesthesia using dorsal penile nerve block, 1 cc of 1% lidocaine without epinephrine
EBL: minimal.
Indications for procedure: Parent desired newborn circumcision of their male infant. Prior to the procedure, the infant was examined and has no signs of hypospadias or illness.
Risks, benefits, alternatives: Were discussed with the parent prior to the procedure, and informed consent was obtained. Signed consent form is in the infant's medical record. Discussion included, but was not limited to: no medical necessity for the procedure, possible bleeding, infection, damage to the penis or adjacent organs, possible poor cosmetic result and possible need for repeat procedure. All their questions were answered.
Complications: none.
Procedure: Area was prepped and draped in sterile fashion. Local anesthesia was administered as documented above under Anesthesia. After allowing sufficient time for the anesthesia to take effect, circumcision was performed in the usual sterile fashion using a 1.3 cm Gomco clamp. Good cosmesis and hemostasis was obtained. Vaseline gauze was applied. Infant tolerated the procedure well. Mother was instructed how to care for the circumcision site.

,.circumcision-mogen

Procedure: Infant circumcision using the Mogen clamp
Anesthesia using Ring block, 1 cc of 1% lidocaine without epinephrine
EBL: minimal.
Indications for procedure: Parent desired newborn circumcision of their male infant. Prior to the procedure, the infant was examined and has no signs of hypospadias or illness.
Risks, benefits, alternatives were discussed with the parent prior to the procedure, and informed consent was obtained. Signed consent form is in the infant's medical record. Discussion included, but was not limited to no medical necessity for the procedure, possible bleeding, infection, damage to the penis or adjacent organs, possible poor cosmetic result and possible need for repeat procedure. All their questions were answered.
Complications: none.

Procedure: Area was prepped and draped in sterile fashion. Local anesthesia was administered as documented above under Anesthesia. After allowing sufficient time for the anesthesia to take effect, circumcision was performed in the usual sterile fashion using a Mogen clamp. Good cosmesis and hemostasis was obtained. Vaseline gauze was applied. Infant tolerated the procedure well. Mother was instructed how to care for the circumcision site.

,.down-sd

Accompanied by caregiver - parent.
Some cognitive disability.
Reports language delay.
Some verbal and nonverbal communication impairment.
No behavioral difficulties.
Pt has a routine for daily activities.
Requires family support.
Community support:
Doing well at school.
Denies anxiety or depression.
Chronic constipation.
No h/o hypothyroidism.
No known h/o cardiovascular ds or VSD.

,.down-sd#

Down Syndrome
Verbal and cognitive capacity, moderate impairment.
Good educational/activity, continue daily routine.
Family and social support: adequate.

,.hand-foot-mouth-ds-PE

Multiple painful 1-3 mm vesicles, some ulcerated and erythematous background involving perioral, bilateral hands and feet. Oral mucosa not involved.

,.obesity-childhood#

Childhood Obesity
Discussed appropriate weight for age.
Goal of losing 1 lb per month.
Discussed 5210 behavioral changes.
Encouraged/praised to build confidence.

,.sports-physical

Here for routine sports physical exam.
Has never been denied or restricted from participation in sports for any reason.
Denies any medical conditions such as asthma, anemia, diabetes or skin infections.
Denies family history of cardiac ds or sudden cardiac death.
Does not take any medications.
NKDA.
No recent illnesses, no GI complaints, denies headaches or fatigue.
No recent hospitalizations or surgeries.
Regular diet, not a lot of junk food. Good appetite.
No recent excessive weight gain or loss.
No vision or hearing changes.
Denies experimenting with cigarettes, alcohol or street drugs.
No smokers at home.
Not sexually active.
Doing well in school; good student.
Wishes to participate in _.

,.sports-physical#

Sports Physical
Cleared for all sports participation without restriction.
Vision screen: _. Un/corrected.
Hgb: WNL.
UA: WNL.

Counseling:.
Diet – balanced diet, avoid junk food.
Accident prevention – bike helmet, risk taking behavior.
Guidance – smoking, alcohol, drugs. peer pressure. regular exercise. academic activities.

Return for next WCC.

,.sports-physical-PE

General: well nourished and developed. No obvious Marfan stigmata. No abuse/neglect evident.
Head: no lesions.
Eyes: PERRL, conjunctivae, sclera clear.
Ears: Canals clear, TMs normal. No cauliflower ear. Normal hearing.
Nose: Passages clear, no lesions.
Teeth: normal dentition.
Neck: Supple, no masses, no thyromegaly. No LAD.
Chest: Symmetrical.
Heart: No murmurs. Regular rhythm.
Lungs: Clear to auscultation.
Abdomen: Soft, no masses, no tenderness, no organomegaly.
 Genitalia: Grossly normal, normal development.
   Male: Testes down, no lesions or masses. No inguinal hernias.
Extremities: No deformities, full range of motion, no edema, pulses strong and equal.
Skin: Clear, no lesions.
Neurologic: alert, physiological. CN 2-12 WNL.
Psych: Appropriate affect with appropriate conversation.

Musculoskeletal: no scoliosis. Full range of motion. Equal strength and mobility of major joint and muscle groups.

,.wcc-mo-0-1

Here for WCC.
Birth history: born at term, NSVD.
Pregnancy complications: none.
Birth weight: _.
Prenatal complications: none.
Interval history: as above
Feedings: breast-feeding every 2-3 hours.
Stools: after each meal.
Cord: present/fell
Circumcision: no.
Infant sleeping position: back.
Exposure to tobacco smoke: no.
Growth and development:
Prone, lifts head briefly.
Moro reflex present.
Turns head side to side.
Blinks at bright light.
Responds to sound.

,.wcc-mo-0-1#

Well child exam.

Nutritional assessment made.
Counseling:
Diet – breast vs. formula feeding, burping, no other p.o. intake, no bottle recumbent.
Behavior – feeding, sleeping, crying, hiccoughs, stools, sneezing.
Accident prevention – falls, ability to roll, smoke detector, burns from hot liquids.

Guidance – spoiling, sibling relationships, diaper rash, circumcision care, cord care, suctioning, pacifier, smoking at home, stimulating with hanging objects and bright colors, thermometer use, call MD for fever.
Infant car seat, crib safety reviewed.

f/u for 2 mo WCC.

,.wcc-mo-01-2

Here for WCC.
Interval history: no interim relevant events.
Diet: Breast-feeding.
Illnesses: none.
Stools: after each meal.
Meds/vitamins: none.
Accidents: none.
Sleep pattern: up to 16 to 17 hours a day. two to four hours at a time.
Exposure to tobacco smoke: none.
Growth/development:
Prone, lifts head 45deg.
Vocalizes (cooing).
Smiles responsively (social).
Follows past midline.
Kicks.
Grasps.

,.wcc-mo-01-2#

Well child exam.

DTaP#1 given. (Pediarix)
HepB#2 given. (Pediarix)
IPV#1 given. (Pediarix)
Rota#1 given.
HiB#1 given.
PCV#1 given.

Vaccine reactions, risks and follow-up explained.

Nutritional assessment made.
Counseling:
Diet – breast vs. formula feeding, no milk or honey till 1 y/o, no bottle recumbent, feeding position, colic.
Behavior – crying, thumb sucking, no discipline yet.
Accident prevention – rolling, playpen use, burns from hot liquids.
Guidance – fever, acetaminophen dose, hot water temp 120deg F, ABCD's to hear, smoking at home.
Safety precautions – infant car seat, water safety, falls, nursery equipment.
Parental smoking discussed.
Childcare plan reviewed.
Emergency care plan reviewed.
Sibling and family relationships discussed.
Thermometer use reviewed.
Umbilical care reviewed.
Infant care (bathing, skin, clothing) reviewed.

f/u for 4 mo WCC

,.wcc-mo-03-4

Here for WCC.
Interval history: no interim relevant events.
Diet: Breast-feeding, formula supplementation.
Illnesses: none.
Stools: no constipation.
Meds/vitamins: none.
Accidents: no.
Sleep pattern: up to 16 to 17 hours a day. two to four hours at a time.
Exposure to tobacco smoke: no.
Growth/development:
Head steady when sitting.
Eyes follow 180deg.
Grasps rattle.
Rolls side to side.

Squeals or goos.
Orients to voices.

,.wcc-mo-03-4#

Well child exam.

Rota#2 given.
DTaP#2 given.
Hib#2 given.
PCV#2 given.
IPV#2 given.
Vaccine reactions, risks and follow-up explained.

Nutritional assessment made.
Counseling:
Diet – breast vs. formula feeding, no milk or honey till 1 y/o, no bottle recumbent, feeding position, colic.
Behavior – rolling, reaching for objects.
Accident prevention – rolling, playpen use, burns from hot liquids.
Guidance – teething, no bottle recumbent, URI treatment, aspiration risk with small objects, language stimulation, no discipline yet.
Safety precautions – infant car seat, water safety, falls, nursery equipment, smoke detector, hot water temp, choking prevention.
Childcare plan reviewed.
Emergency care plan reviewed.
Sibling and family relationships discussed.
Thermometer use reviewed.
Minor illness care reviewed.
Umbilical care reviewed.
Infant care (bathing, skin, clothing) reviewed.
Family spacing discussed.

f/u for 6 mo WCC

,.wcc-mo-05-6

Here for WCC.
Interval history: no interim relevant events.
Diet: Breast-feeding, formula supplementation.
Illnesses: none.
Stools: no constipation.
Meds/vitamins: none.
Accidents: no.
Sleep pattern: several naps, more night-time sleep.
Exposure to tobacco smoke: no.
Growth/development:
No head lag when pulled to sitting.
Reaches for objects.
Bears weight on legs.
Orients to bell.
Rolls both ways.
Sits briefly alone.
Gums, teethes objects.
Babbles.

,.wcc-mo-05-6#

Well child exam.

   DTaP#3 given. (Pediarix)
   HepB#3 given. (Pediarix)
   IPV#3 given. (Pediarix)
   Rota#3 given.
   HiB#3 given.
   PCV#3 given.
   Vaccine reactions, risks and follow-up explained.

Nutritional assessment made.
Counseling:
  Diet – intro solids at 5 mos (rice cereal, vegs, fruit), solids 1 new/week, start with iron-rich, no milk yet, breastfeeding, formula.
  Behavior – begins to sit and crawl, discrimination of people.

Accident prevention – smoke detector, poisoning risk, drug and toxic chemical storage, poison center phone number, childproofing: safety gates, pool fence, hot liquids and surfaces, hot water temp, choking prevention.

Guidance – consistent sleep schedule, teething, blocks, repetitive games, no bottle recumbent, parent smoking.
Infant vs. toddler car seat discussed.
Infant care (bathing, skin, clothing) reviewed.
Childcare plan reviewed.

f/u for 9 mo WCC

,.wcc-mo-07-9

Here for WCC.
Interval history: no interim relevant events.
Diet: introduced solids.
Illnesses: none.
Stools: no constipation.
Meds/vitamins: none.
Accidents: no
Sleep pattern: few naps, more night-time sleep.
Exposure to tobacco smoke: no.
Growth/development:
Sits without support.
Feeds self cracker.
Transfer objects hand to hand.
Mama, dada indiscriminately.
Begins to creep and crawl.
Looks for toys dropped.
Teeth.

,.wcc-mo-07-9#

Well child exam.
  Hct done.
  Vaccines UTD.

Counseling:
   Diet – mashed table food, finger foods, start cup.
   Behavior – sitting, crawling, creeping, trying to pull self up.
   Accident prevention – no food chunks or hard objects the size of a baby's pinky, smoke detector, poisoning risk, drug and toxic chemical storage, poison center phone no., burns: hot liquids and foods, water / pool safety.
   Guidance – decrease in appetite, understands "no" but not discipline, brush teeth, no bottle recumbent.
   Toddler car seats >20lbs.
   Teething problems reviewed.
   Dental hygiene discussed.
Childcare plan reviewed.

f/u for 12 mo WCC

,.wcc-mo-10-12

Here for WCC.
Interval history: no interim relevant events.
Diet: table food.
Illnesses: none.
Stools: no constipation.
Meds/vitamins: none.
Accidents: no.
Sleep pattern: couple naps, more night-time sleep.
Exposure to tobacco smoke: no.
Growth/development:
Pulls self to standing.
Stands holding on.
Holds cup to drink.
Dada, mama.
Thumb-finger grasp.
Plays pat-a-cake.
Walks with help.
Scribbles.

,.wcc-mo-10-12#

Well child exam.

HepB#3 given.
HIB#4 given.
PCV#4 given.
IPV#4 given.
MMR#1 given.
Var#1 given.
HepA#1 given.

Labs: sent for CBC and Lead.

Nutritional assessment made.

Counseling:
Diet – intro meats and proteins, mashed table food, finger foods, start feeder cup, milk, junk food, weaning, normal decreased appetite.
Behavior – minor discipline, pulls to standing.
Accident prevention – no hard objects the size of baby's pinky, smoke detector, drug and toxic chemical storage, poison center phone no., childproofing: electrical outlet covers, safety gates, pool fence, hot liquids and surfaces, hot water temp., drowning, gun in home, falls, walkers, stairs.
Guidance – allow to feed self, look in mirror, play with cloth book, expect growth and appetite to decrease.
Toddler car seats.
Childcare plan reviewed.

f/u for 15 mo WCC

,.wcc-mo-13-15

Here for WCC.
Interval history: no interim relevant events.
Diet: table food.
Illnesses: none.
Stools: no constipation.

Meds/vitamins: none.
Accidents: no.
Sleep pattern: couple naps, sleeps most of the night.
Exposure to tobacco smoke: no.
Growth/development:
Walks alone well.
Takes lid off containers.
Dada, mama, specific.
3 word vocabulary.
Feeds self.
Plays pat-a-cake.
Stoops and recovers.
Scribbles.
2 block tower.

,.wcc-mo-13-15#

Well child exam.

HepB#3 given.
DTaP#4 given.
HIB#4 given.
PCV#4 given.
IPV#4 given.
MMR#1 given.
Var#1 given.
HepA#1 given.

Nutritional assessment made.

Counseling:
Diet – table food, milk, junk food, using cup/bottle, encourage solids.
Behavior – feeding self, simple games.
Accident prevention – no hard objects the size of baby's pinky, smoke detector, drug and toxic chemical storage, poison center phone no., childproofing: safety gates, pool fence, hot liquids and surfaces, hot water

temp., drowning, gun in home, home first aid kit, matches, cabinets and latches.
   Guidance – explain temper tantrums, not ready for toilet training, bottle, toothbrush.
Toddler car seats.
Childcare plan reviewed.
Emergency care plan reviewed.

f/u for 18 mo WCC

,.wcc-mo-16-23

Here for WCC.
Interval history: no interim relevant events.
Diet: table food.
Illnesses: none.
Stools: no constipation.
Meds/vitamins: none.
Accidents: no.
Sleep pattern: couple naps, sleeps through the night.
Exposure to tobacco smoke: no.
Growth/development:
Walks alone well.
Takes lid off containers.
Dada, mama, specific.
3 word vocabulary.
Feeds self.
Plays pat-a-cake.
Stoops and recovers.
Scribbles.
2 block tower.

,.wcc-mo-16-23#

Well child exam.

Vaccines are UTD.

Nutritional assessment made.

Counseling:
Diet – regular meals with snacks, cup only: no bottle (12-15mos), junk food.
Behavior – runs but falls easily, loves rough play.
Accident prevention – no hard objects the size of baby's pinky, smoke detector, drug and toxic chemical storage, poison center phone no., childproofing: safety gates, pool fence, hot liquids and surfaces, hot water hemp., drowning, gun in home, falls from chairs.
Guidance – reading to child, toilet awareness not training, toothbrush use, parent smoking.
Toddler car seats.
Childcare plan reviewed.
Emergency care plan reviewed.

f/u for 2 yr WCC

,.wcc-pe-infant

General: well nourished and developed.
No abuse/neglect evident.
Head: no lesions.
Eyes: PERRL, conjunctivae, sclera clear. + Red reflex bilat.
Ears: Canals clear, TMs normal.
Nose: Passages clear, no lesions.
Teeth: grossly normal.
Neck: Supple, no masses, no thyromegaly.
Chest: Symmetrical.
Heart: No organic murmurs, regular rhythm.
Lungs: Clear to auscultation.
Abdomen: Soft, no masses, no tenderness, no organomegaly.
Hips: Good abduction, no hip click noted.
Genitalia: Grossly normal, normal development.
    Male: Testes down, no lesions.

Extremities: No deformities, full range of motion.
Femoral pulses: normal.
Lymph nodes: not enlarged.
Back: No scoliosis.
Skin: Clear, no significant lesions.
Neurologic: alert, physiological.

,.wcc-pe-pub/teen

General: well nourished and developed.
No abuse/neglect evident.
Head: no lesions.
Eyes: PERRL, conjunctivae, sclera clear. + Red reflex bilat.
Ears: Canals clear, TMs normal.
Nose: Passages clear, no lesions.
Teeth: grossly normal.
Neck: Supple, no masses, no thyromegaly.
Chest: Symmetrical.
Heart: No organic murmurs, regular rhythm.
Lungs: Clear to auscultation.
Abdomen: Soft, no masses, no tenderness, no organomegaly.
Genitalia: Grossly normal, normal development.
  Male: Testes down, no lesions.
    Tanner stage:
    [Genital
      1. Prepubertal
      2. Normal size testicles
      3. Penis enlargement
      4. Penis increased breadth
     Pubic Hair
      1. Prepubertal
      2. Fine hair
      3. Curly hair.
      4. Complete fulled triangle
      5. hair spreads to medial aspect of thighs
     Breast
      1. prepubertal

2. BReast lumps/buds
   3. Elevated Areola
   4. Separation of breast
   5. Total breast development]
Extremities: No deformities, full range of motion.
Back: No scoliosis.
Skin: Clear, no significant lesions.
Neurologic: alert, physiological.

,.wcc-pe-toddler/child

General: well nourished and developed.
No abuse/neglect evident.
Head: no lesions.
Eyes: PERRL, conjunctivae, sclera clear. + Red reflex bilat.
Ears: Canals clear, TMs normal.
Nose: Passages clear, no lesions.
Teeth: grossly normal.
Neck: Supple, no masses, no thyromegaly.
Chest: Symmetrical.
Heart: No organic murmurs, regular rhythm.
Lungs: Clear to auscultation.
Abdomen: Soft, no masses, no tenderness, no organomegaly.
Genitalia: Grossly normal, normal development.
   Male: Testes down, no lesions.
Extremities: No deformities, full range of motion.
Lymph nodes: not enlarged.
Back: No scoliosis.
Skin: Clear, no significant lesions.
Neurologic: alert, physiological.

,.wcc-yrs-02

Here for WCC.
Interval history: no relevant interim events.
Diet: breakfast: _, lunch: _, dinner: _, snacks: _.

Illnesses: none.
Stools: no constipation.
Meds/vitamins: none.
Accidents: no.
Sleep pattern: couple naps, sleeps through the night.
Screen time: <2 hours.
Exposure to tobacco smoke: no.
Growth/development:
Runs well, walks up and down.
Identified 1 body part.
Kicks and throws a ball.
7-20 word vocabulary.
Puts on simple clothes.
Puts 2-3 words together.
Handles spoon well.
Plays hide and seek.
3 block tower.
Helps in house.

,.wcc-yrs-02#

Well child exam.

Vaccines are UTD.

Hct done.
UA done.
Nutritional assessment made.
Counseling:.
Diet – regular meals with snacks, iron-rich foods, sodium, caloric balance, switch to lowfat milk.   Tap water.
Behavior – Disciple, tantrums, time out, imitates .
Accident prevention – street dangers, falls, drowning, poison center, storage of drugs, toxic chemicals, guns, smoke detectors, hot water temp, pool fence, bike helmet.

Guidance – start toilet training, parallel peer play, monitor TV programs, brush teeth, dentist q1-2 years, effects of passive smoking, protect skin from UV light.
Toddler car seat.
Childcare plan reviewed.
Emergency care plan reviewed.

f/u for 3 yr WCC

,.wcc-yrs-03

Here for WCC.
Interval history: no relevant interim events.
Diet: breakfast: _, lunch: _, dinner: _, snacks: _.
Illnesses: none.
Stools: no constipation.
Meds/vitamins: none.
Accidents: no.
Sleep pattern: naps, 10 hrs at night.
Screen time: <2 hours.
Exposure to tobacco smoke: no.
Growth/development:
Goes up stairs alternating feet.
Plays with other children.
Knows age, sex, first and last name.
Balance on each foot, 1 second.
Vocabulary of about 500 words.
Helps in dressing.
Copies +.
20 teeth.
Cuts with scissors.

,.wcc-yrs-03#

Well child exam.

Vaccines are UTD.

Hct done.
Vision screening.
Audiometry.
Nutritional assessment made.
Dental referral.

Counseling:

Diet – regular meals with snacks, caloric balance, sweets, iron. Tap water.
Behavior – model appropriate language, praise good behavior, encourage self-expression of feelings (anger/sadness/frustration), very aware of peers.
Accident prevention – street dangers, knives, falls, drowning, caution with strangers, smoke detectors, hot water temp, pool fence, play equipment, bike helmet, poison center phone, storage of drugs, toxic chemicals, guns.
Guidance – read together, TV programs, regular exercise, brush teeth, dentist q1-2 years, UV skin protection, parent smoking.
Toddler car seat till 4 years and under 40 lbs.
Childcare plan reviewed.
Emergency care plan reviewed.

f/u for 4 yr WCC

,.wcc-yrs-04-5

Here for WCC.
Interval history: no relevant interim events.
Diet: breakfast: _, lunch: _, dinner: _, snacks: _.
Illnesses: none.
Stools: no constipation.
Meds/vitamins: none.
Accidents: no.
Sleep pattern: naps, 10 hrs at night.
Screen time: <2 hours.
Exposure to tobacco smoke: no.
Growth/development:

Hops on one foot.
Counts 4 pennies.
Copies a square.
Catches, throws a ball.
Plays with several children.
Recognizes 3-4 colors.
Knows opposites.
Knows name, address, phone number.

,.wcc-yrs-04-5#

Well child exam.

DTaP given.
IPV given.
MMR given.
VAR given.

Hct done.
UA done.
Vision screening.
Audiometry.
Nutritional assessment made.
Dental referral.

Counseling:

Diet – regular meals with snacks, caloric balance, sweets, iron. Tap water.
Behavior – model appropriate language, praise good behavior, encourage self-expression of feelings (anger/sadness/frustration), very aware of peers.
Accident prevention – street dangers, falls, drowning, caution with strangers, smoke detectors, hot water temp, window guards, pool fence, play equipment, bike helmet, poison center phone, storage of drugs, toxic chemicals, matches, guns.
Guidance – knows name, address and phone no., plays with other children, imitates adults, dressing self, brushing own teeth, school plans, TV

programs, regular exercise, UV skin protection, dentist q1-2 yrs, parent smoking.
Seat belt use.
Childcare plan reviewed.
Emergency care plan reviewed.

f/u for 5/6 yr WCC

,.wcc-yrs-06-8

Here for WCC.
Interval history: no relevant interim events.
Diet: breakfast: _, lunch: _, dinner: _, snacks: _.
Illnesses: none.
Weight loss/gain: not significant.
Stools: no constipation.
Illnesses, stomach, headache, fatigue: no.
Fatigue, nightmares, enuresis: no.
Meds/vitamins: none.
Accidents: no.
Sleep pattern: naps, 10 hrs at night.
Screen time: <2 hours.
Exposure to tobacco smoke: no.
Growth/school progress (achievement, sports, peer relationships, attendance, school vision or hearing problems): no.
Balances on 1 foot.
Dances, swims, rides a bicycle.
Knows left from right .
Like table/ board games.
Prints numbers to 10.
Other- prints first name, draws person with 6 parts.

,.wcc-yrs-06-8#

Well child exam.

DTaP given.
IPV given.
MMR given.
VAR given.

Hct done.
UA done.
Vision screening.
Audiometry.
Nutritional assessment made.
Dental referral.

Counseling:

Diet – limit sweets, sodium, fat (esp sat + chol), snacks, balanced meals.
Accident prevention – bike helmet, water safety, car safety, smoke detector, storage of guns, drugs, toxic chemicals, matches.
Guidance – bed time, discipline, tooth brushing, dentist q1-2 years, UV skin protection, regular exercise, school achievement, fun, friends, family life education, child sexual abuse.
Seat belt use.

f/u for next WCC or prn.

,.wcc-yrs-09-12

Here for WCC.
Interval history: no relevant interim events.
Diet: breakfast: _, lunch: _, dinner: _, snacks: _.
Appetite: good.
Physical activity: frequent.
Weight loss/gain: no.
Stools: no constipation.
Illnesses, stomach, headache, fatigue: no.
Meds/vitamins: none.
Accidents: no.
Sleep pattern: naps, 10 hrs at night.

Screen time: <2 hours.
Exposure to tobacco smoke: no.

HEADSS
Lives @ home. Safe environment.
Attends _th grade. Doing ok at school. Grades: (A/B). Not currently employed.
Activities: Plays _.
Denies using tobacco/alcohol/drugs. No pressure from peers.
Not sexually active.
Denies any depression symptoms. Not suicidal.

,.wcc-yrs-09-12#

Well child exam.

Hct done.
UA done.
Nutritional assessment made.
Dental referral.
Vision screening.
Audiometry.

MMR#2 given.
Td given.
Varicella given.
HepB vax given.
Gardasil vax given.

Additional labs: .

Counseling:.
Diet – limit sweets, sodium, fat (esp sat + chol), snacks, balanced meals.
Tap water.
Accident prevention – bike helmet, water safety, car safety, smoke detector, storage of guns, drugs, toxic chemicals.

Guidance – bed time, discipline, smoking, alcohol, marijuana, cocaine, IV and other drugs, family life education, early sex education and puberty progress, exercise 3 times a week, health decisions, TV, school, fun, friends, UV light protection, tooth brushing, dentist yearly, sexual abuse, violence prevention.
Seat belt use.

f/u for next WCC or prn

,.wcc-yrs-13-16

Here for WCC.
Interval history: no relevant interim events.
Diet: breakfast: _, lunch: _, dinner: _, snacks: _.
Appetite: good.
Physical activity: frequent.
Weight loss/gain: no.
Stools: no constipation.
Illnesses, stomach, headache, fatigue: no.
Meds/vitamins: none.
Accidents: no.
Sleep pattern: naps, 10 hrs at night.
Screen time: <2 hours.
Exposure to tobacco smoke: no.

HEADSS
Lives @ home. Safe environment.
Attends _th grade. Doing ok at school. Grades: (A/B). Not currently employed.
Activities: Plays _.
Denies using tobacco/alcohol/drugs. No pressure from peers.
Not sexually active.
Denies any depression symptoms. Not suicidal.

„.wcc-yrs-13-16#

Well child exam.

Hct done.
UA done.
Nutritional assessment made.
Dental referral.
Vision screening.
Audiometry.
GC/Chlamydia: done. Not sexually active. Refused.

MMR#2 given.
Td given.
Varicella given.
HepB vax given.
Gardasil vax given.

Additional labs: .

Counseling:.
Diet – healthy diet, caloric balance, appropriate weight, junk food, eating disorders. Tap water.
Accident prevention – bike helmet, risk taking behavior, DUI, guns, violent behavior, motor vehicle safety, work safety.
Guidance – smoking, alcohol, marijuana, cocaine, IV and other drugs, depression, suicidal ideation, puberty progress, sex education (partner selection, condoms, contraception, AIDS risk factors), goals in life, family interaction.
Seat belt use.
Personal development: physical, growth, sexuality, independence.

f/u for next WCC or prn

„.wcc-yrs-17-18

Here for WCC.
Interval history: no relevant interim events.

Diet: breakfast: _, lunch: _, dinner: _, snacks: _.
Appetite: good.
Physical activity: frequent.
Weight loss/gain: no.
Stools: no constipation.
Illnesses, stomach, headache, fatigue: no.
Meds/vitamins: none.
Accidents: no.
Sleep pattern: naps, 10 hrs at night.
Screen time: <2 hours.
Exposure to tobacco smoke: no.

HEADSS
Lives @ home. Safe environment.
Attends _th grade. Doing ok at school. Grades: (A/B). Not currently employed.
Activities: Plays _.
Denies using tobacco/alcohol/drugs. No pressure from peers.
Not sexually active.
Denies any depression symptoms. Not suicidal.

,.wcc-yrs-17-18#

Well child exam.

Hct done.
UA done.
Nutritional assessment made.
Dental referral.
Vision screening.
Audiometry.
GC/Chlamydia: done. Not sexually active. Refused.

MMR#2 given.
Td given.
Varicella given.
HepB vax given.

Gardasil vax given.

Additional labs: none.

Counseling:.
Diet – obesity, eating disorders, junk food. Tap water.
Accident prevention – bike helmet, risk taking behavior, DUI, guns, violent behavior, motor vehicle safety, work safety.
Guidance – smoking, alcohol, marijuana, cocaine, IV and other drugs, depression, suicidal ideation, puberty progress, sex education (partner selection, condoms, contraception, AIDS risk factors), goals in life, regular exercise.
Seat belt use reviewed.
Personal development, independence discussed.
Academic, work activities reviewed.
Family, social interaction, communication discussed.

f/u for next WCC or prn

,.wt+bili-check

Here for wt and bili check.
Born at term via repeat LTCS, no complications.
Birth wt: _3409 g.
Breast and bottle feeding.
Normal stool and voiding pattern.
No interim events.

,.wt+bili-check#

Wt and bili check
Exam WNL.
<_8% wt loss.
Bili _low-risk level.
Encouraged continue breastfeeding.

Precautions given for decreased PO intake, decreased wet diapers, fever>100.4.
F/u in 2 wks for WCC.

,.wt+bili-check-PE

General: Awake and alert. No acute distress.
Eye: Normal conjunctiva. No ictericia.
Integumentary: Warm. Pink. No jaundice.

13 PSYCHOLOGY

,.adhd

Patient c/o symptoms of inattention, impulsivity, and restlessness, resulting in functional impairment.
Reports symptoms since being adolescent.
No attention to details, difficulty sustaining attention, does not follow instructions, forgetful.
Often fidgets, unable to engage in leisure activities quietly, talks excessively, interrupts, difficulty waiting for his turn.

,.adhd#

ADHD
Discussed behavioral therapy.
 Exercise after school.
 Healthy diet.
 Decrease screen time <2 hrs.
 Sleep hygiene.
 Mindful meditation.
Consider IEP. Parent will ask at school.
Recommended community resources.
Recommended book for parent education (The nurtured heart approach).

Gave Parent/Teacher Vanderbilt assessment. Will bring back at next visit. Will consider stimulant tx if dx confirmed and no improvement w/ behavioral tx.

,.adhd#-adult

ADHD, adult
Adult ADHD Self-Report Scale (ASRS-v1.1) Symptom Checklist highly consistent with diagnosis.
Discussed behavioral therapy.
Exercise.
Healthy diet.
Decrease screen time <2 hrs.
Sleep hygiene.
Mindful meditation.
Will consider stimulant tx if dx confirmed and no improvement w/ behavioral tx.

,.adhd#-f/u

ADHD
Stable.
Continue behavioral therapy.
Continue current stimulant dose.

,.adhd-f/u

ADHD
Patient reports good control of symptoms of inattention, impulsivity, and restlessness,
On stimulant. Compliant with meds. Denies any side effects.
Enables pt to have a functional professional life.

,.adhd-letter

Dear principal,

The above named student was diagnosed with attention deficit hyperactivity disorder (ADHD). By this office on _ and was last seen on _. The diagnosis was based on patient, family and teacher reports, physical examination, diagnostic criteria, standardized questionnaires, and other testing. Medical and behavioral treatment and monitoring will be ongoing.

Although our evaluation focused on ADHD we also discussed with the parents learning and behavior disorders, school-based educational/behavioral assessments, section 504, IDEA, and psychometric academic/achievement testing. Information given to the parents included "educational rights for children with ADHD" at http://www.help4adhd.org.

This medical report documents that a diagnosis of ADHD, a neurobiological disorder which may limit learning thereby qualifying the student for appropriate academic or behavioral accommodations. Modifications recommended by section 504 of the rehabilitation act of 1973 include "physical arrangement of room, lesson preparation, assignments/worksheets, transportation, test-taking, organization, behaviors, medications, discipline or other as specified."

This letter is a formal request from the parents and the physician for further psychological and academic assessments of this student. A copy of this notification has been given to the parent for their use and is on file in our medical records department.

Thank you for this opportunity to work cooperatively with you and my patient's family.

Sincerely,

,.adhd-letter-adult

To Whom It May Concern,

The above named student was diagnosed with attention deficit hyperactivity disorder (ADHD). By this office on _ and was last seen on _. The diagnosis was based on patient and family reports, physical examination, diagnostic criteria, standardized questionnaires, and other testing. Medical and behavioral treatment and monitoring will be ongoing.

Although our evaluation focused on ADHD we also discussed with the patient learning and behavior disorders, school-based educational/ behavioral assessments, section 504, IDEA, and psychometric academic/ achievement testing. Information given to the parents included "educational rights for people with ADHD" at http://www.help4adhd.org.

This medical report documents that a diagnosis of ADHD, a neurobiological disorder which may limit learning thereby qualifying the student for appropriate academic or behavioral accommodations. Modifications recommended by section 504 of the rehabilitation act of 1973 include "physical arrangement of room, lesson preparation, assignments/worksheets, transportation, test-taking, organization, behaviors, medications, discipline or other as specified."

Thank you for this opportunity to work cooperatively with you and this patient.

Sincerely,

,.anxiety

Anxiety
Experiencing physical and emotional stress.
Complains of life stressors, feels stressed about _.
Excessive worrying about _.
Symptoms have been present for >6 months. Impairing sleep and concentration.
Complains of fatigue and irritability. No CP, SOB, GI symptoms.
No history of physical or emotional trauma or death of a loved one.
Does not report panic attacks.

Denies any use of drugs, excessive caffeine or alcohol. No thyroid disease.
No Family Hx of psychiatric conditions.
Endorses depression. Denies suicidal ideation.
Denies any manic or hypomanic episodes.
Denies any visual or auditory hallucinations.

,.anxiety#

Anxiety
Start Continue SSRIs.
Recommended Cognitive Behavioral Therapy.
Reviewed relaxation techniques.
Recommended mindfulness meditation and exercise. Sleep hygiene.
Insight-oriented psychotherapy given for 16 minutes exclusively.
Psychoeducation: encouraged personality growth and development through coping techniques and problem-solving skills.

,.anxiety-f/u

Anxiety
Compliant with SSRI. no side effects.
Not attending psychotherapy.
Experiencing less physical and emotional stress.
Exercising.
Sleeping more than 6 hrs.
Does not report panic attacks.
No CP, SOB, GI symptoms or palpitations.
Denies depression or suicidal ideation.

,.autism

Autism
Reports no language delay.
No verbal or nonverbal communication impairment.
No social impairment.

No repetitive behavior, no stereotyped interest.
Pt has a routine for daily activities.
Requires family support.
Community support:
Doing well at school.
Does not have an Individual Education Program.
No sleeping difficulties.
Denies anxiety or depression.

,.autism#

Autism
Verbal and cognitive capacity, close to normal.
Monitor educational progress, seems to have appropriate education at this point.
Family support: referred to local support resources.

,.binge-eating

Binge eating
Patient reports struggling with the amount of food eaten.
Reports lack of control and distress over eating.
These episodes occur more than once a week.
Patient reports low self-esteem and depression over the situation and inability to lose weight.

,.binge-eating#

Binge eating disorder
Cognitive behavioral therapy. Referred to psychotherapy.
Started SSRI.

,.bipolar-ds

Bipolar disorder
On no meds.
No recent manic episodes.
A few episodes of depression during last year.
No suicidal ideation.

,.bipolar-ds#

Bipolar disorder
Stable w/o recent acute episodes.
Continue current management without changes.
Psychosocial interventions and monitoring.

,.borderline

BPD
Pt endorses
 Emotional instability and unpredictable outbursts.
 Impulsivity.
 Intense, unstable, and conflicted interpersonal relationships.
 Disturbed self-image, aims, and preferences.
 Chronic feelings of emptiness.
 Tendency for self-destructive behavior, including suicide gestures and behavior.

,.borderline#

Borderline personality disorder
Dx confirmed with MacLean Screening Instrument for BPD.
Recommended Cognitive Behavioral Therapy.
Bibliotherapy.

,.bulimia

Bulimia
Pt reports recurrent episodes of binge eating with compensatory vomiting.
Started with behavior a year ago, but worsening in the last 3 months.
Concerned about weight and body shape.
Endorses palpitations and sore throat.
Endorses fluctuation in weight.
+ anxiety and depression.

,.buprenorphine

Opioid use disorder
On buprenorphine.
Denies any side effects like sedation, headaches, nausea, constipation or insomnia.
Does not use any benzodiazepines or alcohol.

,.buprenorphine#

Opioid use disorder
On buprenorphine. Stable.
Continue current management per psych.

,.bulimia#

Bulimia
Cognitive behavioral therapy. Referred to psychotherapy.
Nutrition and meal support. Referred to nutritionist.
Started fluoxetine.

,.depression

Depression

Compliant with SSRI. No side effects.
Not attending psychotherapy.
Denies feeling depressed or having little interest in doing things.
No suicidal ideations.

,.depression#

Depression
Stable. Continue SSRI without dose changes.
PHQ-9 Score: _ moderate, recurrent.
Reviewed Cognitive Behavioral Therapy.
Recommended mindfulness meditation and exercise. Sleep hygiene.
Ventilation and insight-oriented psychotherapy given for 16 minutes exclusively.
Psychoeducation: encouraged personality growth and development through coping techniques and problem-solving skills.

,.etoh

Not concerned about alcohol problem.
Drinks _ day/week.
Has ~ _ drinks when drinking.
Denies not being able to stop drinking once started.
Not affecting daily life or interfering with responsibilities.
Does not drink an "eye opener".
Denies feeling of guilt/remorse.

Patient does smoke cigarettes.

,.etoh#

Alcohol use disorder
Intervention: Counseled on cessation/cutting down - 15 min.
Patient shows interest.
Feedback about patient's alcohol use.

Psychosocial interventions: Discussed non-pharmacologic tx including CBT, psychotherapy, AA, addiction programs, or other support groups. Consider pharmacotherapy to prevent relapse and support abstinence.

,.etoh/substance-counsel*

99408

,.grief#

Grief
Acute (<1 yr). No other psych/mental ds.
Discussed grief normal response to bereavement.
No tx indicated other than support from family and friends.
Encouraged patient to maintain regular activities, sleep, exercise, and nutrition.
Consider support groups.

,.insomnia

Insomnia
Hours of sleep at night: <6. Naps: no.
Timing: difficulty falling/staying asleep. early awakening.
Daytime effects and symptoms include fatigue.
Sleep schedule/habits: 10-6, TV on.
Sleep environment: dark.
Denies snoring or kicking during the night.
Pt denies any depression or emotional stress.
Does not smoke.
Alcohol: occasional.
No night shift work.

,.insomnia#

Insomnia
CBT. Headspace app.
Reviewed cognitive and behavioral components including:
Sleep hygiene.
Establish bed and wake times.
Sleep restriction. (Only sleep estimated hrs sleep).
Bed only for sex and sleep, only sleep when sleepy, out of bed if anxious (stimulus control).
Reviewed relaxation techniques, mindful meditation.
Expected sleep duration. Addressed worries about not sleeping.

,.insomnia-f/u

Pt c/o persisting insomnia for >3mo.
No depression or anxiety.
No alcohol or tobacco.
Taking medication every night.
Reports improvement in number of hours and sleep quality.

,.methadone

Opioid use disorder
On methadone. Compliant with program.
Denies any side effects like constipation, drowsiness, excessive sweating, swelling, reduced libido or erectile dysfunction.
Does not use any benzodiazepines or alcohol.

,.methadone#

Opioid use disorder
On methadone. Stable.
F/u at methadone clinic.

,.psychotherapy#

Time spent doing psychotherapy exclusive of E/M time: 16 minutes.
Psychotherapy intervention used: Supportive Psychotherapy.

,.psychotx*

90833

,.suboxone

Opioid use disorder
On Suboxone.
Denies any side effects like sedation, headaches, nausea, constipation or insomnia.
Does not use any benzodiazepines or alcohol.

,.suboxone#

Opioid use disorder
On buprenorphine. Stable.
Continue current management per psych.

,.suicide-contract

No-suicide agreement. Pt promises not to do anything to harm or kill herself.
Will contact 911 or go to ED if having suicidal thoughts.
Other resources discussed:
National Suicide Prevention Lifeline - Call 1-800-273-8255 (Available 24 hours everyday).
Lifeline Chat - https://suicidepreventionlifeline.org/chat/

14 PULMONOLOGY

,.asthma

Asthma
On albuterol and Qvar.
SOB/wheezing/use of SABA < 2/week.
Night symptoms < 2/month.
No activity limits.
No hospitalizations for exacerbations during the last year.

,.asthma#

Asthma
Well controlled.
Maintain current tx step.
Explained quick-relief vs controlled meds.
Reviewed inhaler/device technique.
Consider step down if well controlled for >3 mo.
Spirometry done less than a year ago.
Reinforced self monitoring of symptoms and peak flow.

,.asthma-exacerbation

Pt w/ asthma presents with SOB, productive cough and wheezing x days.
Not responding to inhalers.
No fevers or chills.
No URI symptoms.
No sick contacts.

,.asthma-exercise

Asthma
On prn albuterol.
SOB/wheezing only when exercising.
Otherwise no activity limits, no symptoms at night or when at rest.

,.asthma-exercise#

Asthma, exercise induced
Stable.
Continue albuterol prior to exertion.

,.copd

COPD
Compliant with inhalers.
SOB only w/ strenuous exercise/hurrying @ level/walking slight hill.
 SOB w/ walking @ level; must make stops. Productive cough most days.
No hospitalizations for exacerbations during the last year.
Not smoking.

,.copd#

COPD
Well controlled.
-FEV1 >50% of predicted. <2 exacerbations/yr (not hospitalized).

-FEV1 <50% of predicted or >2 exacerbations/yr (or hospitalized).
Continue current inhalers.
No need for O2 tx. O2 Sat>92%, no signs of resp/right heart failure.
Vaccines: flu, pneumococcal. UTD.
Encouraged physical activity.
Spirometry done <1 yr ago.

,.copd-exacerbation

Pt w/ COPD presents with SOB, productive cough and wheezing x days.
No fevers or chills.
No URI symptoms.
No sick contacts.
Not smoking.

,.lung-nodule-incidental

Incidental lung nodule.
Pt is asymptomatic w/o any cough or constitutional symptoms.
Immunocompetent w/o any malignancy that is actively under treatment or follow-up.

,.lung-nodule-incidental#

Incidental lung nodule
Asymptomatic.
Immunocompetent w/o any malignancy.
Size: _ mm.
Per radiology, repeat chest CT in 12 mo.
 Unchanged.
 No further follow-up per radiology.

,.lung-nodule-lung-ca-screen

Lung nodule detected during lung cancer screening.
Pt is asymptomatic w/o any cough or constitutional symptoms.
Not smoking.

,.lung-nodule-lung-ca-screen#

Lung nodule
Detected during lung cancer screening.
Management according to Lung-RADS.
Category: 1
Continue annual screening with LDCT in 12 months.

,.pulmonaryHTN

Pulmonary hypertension
Denies dyspnea or chest pain. No lower extremity swelling.

,.pulmonaryHTN#

Pulmonary hypertension
WHO class III, d/t lung ds and hypoxia.
Asymptomatic w/ ordinary activity.
EF _60-65% (_2013)
On ASA. no need for further anticoagulation.
Stable, monitor.

15 RENAL/UROLOGY

,.balanitis

Pt c/o pain at the tip of penis.
Some difficulty urinating/dysuria.
No itch or penile discharge.
No new partners.
No h/o penile trauma.
No fevers or chills.

,.balanitis#

Balanitis
Improve personal hygiene.
Daily foreskin retraction.
Vinegar and water soaks.
Topical antifungal.
Consider low-potency steroid if not improving.

,.balanitis-PE

Uncircumcised penis, erythema on glans of penis and foreskin.

,.balanitis bxo#

Balanitis xerotica obliterates
Trial of 0.05% clobetasol ointment applied bid until improvement.
Then apply 0.05% betamethasone ointment bid for 1 month.
Very gradual taper off.
Discussed circumcision is curative for phimosis. Consider if no improvement.

,.bph-hpi

BPH
On flomax.
No complains of frequency, nocturia, urgency, incomplete voiding.
No incontinence.

,.bph#

BPH
Mild disease with no significant bother.
Watchful waiting.
Behavioral management (limit fluids, bladder training).

,.bxo#

Balanitis xerotica obliterates
Trial of 0.05% clobetasol ointment applied bid until improvement.
Then apply 0.05% betamethasone ointment bid for 1 month.
Very gradual taper off.
Discussed circumcision is curative for phimosis. Consider if no improvement.

,.ckd-hpi

CKD
Compliant with medications.
Denies peripheral edema, SOB, orthopnea.
Does not check weight at home. Did not notice weight gain.
Patient is not being followed by nephrologist.

,.ckd#

CKD IIIa(GFR45-59) IIIb(GFR30-44)
Stable. No changes in management. Monitor renal function.
Optimal BP and glycemic control. Dietary therapy. Low P and K.
Anemia and bone mineral disorder screen: up-to-date. CMP, P, iPTH.

,.cystitis-int

Interstitial cystitis
Pt c/o urgency, frequency and pelvic-floor pain.
Reports food or stress triggers.

,.cystitis-int#

Interstitial cystitis
Lifestyle changes.
Pelvic physical therapy.
Trial of amitriptyline.

,.erectile-dysfunction

Patient complains of difficulty obtaining/maintaining an erection.
Denies any psychosocial stressors, psychosexual or relationship problems with partner.
Denies any excess alcohol intake.

No history of diabetes, CAD or peripheral arterial disease.
Patient does not smoke.
Denies any premature ejaculation.
Denies any genital pain or numbness.
Patient is not able to obtain erections when awakening.

,.erectile-dysfunction#

Erectile dysfunction
Trial of sildenafil.
Discussed treatment of underlying condition.
Discussed psychosexual therapy.

,.nephrolithiasis

Pt c/o flank pain, left.
Severe, radiates to groin.
Previous episode of nephrolithiasis.
No fever. No N/V. No dysuria.
Denies hematuria.

,.nephrolithiasis#

Renal colic
Recommended hydration, pain control, and prn zofran.
Labs: BMP check renal fx.
UA to check for blood r/o infx.
Medical expulsive therapy with tamsulosin.
Renal US to confirm dx of nephrolithiasis.
If >10 mm or failing med tx refer to urology for sx removal.

,.nephrolithiasis-PE

+ CVA/flank tenderness.

,.oab-hpi

Pt c/o leaking urine when having a strong urge on the way to the bathroom.
Endorses urinary frequency.
Urge to urinate is waking up pt and interfering with sleep.
Has to wear pads for protection.

,.oab#

Overactive bladder
Behavioral approaches + lifestyle changes.
Kegel exercises.
Caffeine reduction, fluid management/reduction.
Trial of antimuscarinics (oxybutynin).Ddiscussed side effects.

,.overactive-bladder

Pt c/o leaking urine when having a strong urge on the way to the bathroom.
Endorses urinary frequency.
Urge to urinate is waking up pt and interfering with sleep.
Has to wear pads for protection.

,.overactive-bladder#

Overactive bladder
Behavioral approaches + lifestyle changes.
Kegel exercises.
Caffeine reduction, fluid management/reduction.
trial of antimuscarinics (oxybutynin). discussed side effects.

,.phimosis

C/o penile partial phimosis.
Some itching.
No painful erections or urination.
No urinary obstruction.

,.phimosis#

Phimosis
Partial.
Not compromising voiding or sexual function.
Consider circumcision.
ED precautions with paraphimosis.

,.phimosis-PE

Penile foreskin with ring atrophy and hypopigmented skin lesion. difficult retraction of glans.

,.ppp-hpi

Pt c/o penile lesions at the tip of his penis.
Present for months.
No new sexual partners.

,.ppp#

Pearly penile papules
Reassured pt.
No tx needed.
Consider laser therapy for cosmetic concerns.

,.ppp-PE

GU: multiple skin-colored, semi-transparent elevated papules arranged in rows on the coronal ring.

,.stress-incontinence

Pt c/o involuntary urine leakage on effort, exertion, sneezing/coughing.
Accompanied by urgency.
Denies any vaginal bulge/pressure sensation.
H/o 3 vaginal deliveries.

,.stress-incontinence#

Stress incontinence
Behavioral approaches + lifestyle changes.
Kegel exercises.
Caffeine reduction, fluid management/reduction.

,.vasectomy*

55250

,.vasectomy-eval

Pt desires not to father any more children.
Has 3 kids.
Interested in male sterilization.
Denies any h/o GU surgeries/scars or trauma.
Denies any chronic medical conditions.

,.vasectomy-eval#

\# Vasectomy evaluation
Procedure and pre/post surgical care discussed with patient.
Discussed this is a permanent procedure, pt expressed understanding.
Consent for sterilization signed.

,.vasectomy-proc

PRE-OP DIAGNOSIS: Desires Elective Sterilization.
POST-OP DIAGNOSIS: Same.
PROCEDURE: Elective Bilateral Vasectomy.
ANESTHESIA: 1:1 mix Lidocaine 1% with and without epi.
Total amount used: 8 mL.

INDICATIONS:
This gentleman desires elective sterilization. He was counseled regarding the risks, alternatives, and benefits of male sterilization by vasectomy. He was informed of the risks of the procedure, including but not limited to failure of the procedure to produce sterility, the risks of bleeding, infection, and injury to scrotal contents. All questions were answered and the required State of California consent form was signed. No guarantees were given or implied. A time out was taken prior to the procedure.

PROCEDURE:
The patient was laid supine on the procedure table. He was sterilely prepped and draped in the usual fashion. The vasa were identified bilaterally. The left vas was grasped using the three-finger technique. Local anesthesia with a 27 gauge needle was applied to the skin in the midline / lateral scrotum and to the left vas and surrounding tissue. A vas fixing forceps was used to grasp the vas through the scrotal skin. A vas dissecting instrument was then used to pierce the skin and down through the fascia. The vas was then identified and delivered through the incision. The surrounding vassal tissue was incised in the midline in a vertical fashion to reveal the vas. The vas was grasped with a vas forceps and delivered out of the fascia. The vas was distally and proximally grasped.

The intervening segment of approximately 2 cm was excised and sent for pathologic review. The lumen of the vas were sealed with thermal fine wire cautery. The proximal vas was then closed over with fascia in a fascial interposition technique.
Small surgical clips were placed on the distal and proximal ends of the vas and.

The right vas was attended to in the same fashion as the left vas after local anesthesia was applied to the vas and surrounding tissue. All bleeding was controlled. The scrotal fascia was allowed to close by primary intention . Sterile dressings were applied and the patient was sent home with standard post-vasectomy instructions, including instructions to take semen sample to the lab for analysis after 15-20 ejaculations.

16 SURGERY

,.abscess

C/o abscess on _.
Present for days.
Became red and painful, worsening.
No spontaneous drainage.
No fever or chills.
No h/o trauma or injury.

,.abscess#

Abscess,
S/p incision and drainage.
The patient tolerated the procedure well without complications.
Standard post-procedure care is explained and return precautions are given.
No antibiotic needed.
Return 1 week for packing replacement and wound care.
Return precautions discussed with patient, including excessive bleeding, fever, worsening of purulent discharge.

,.abscess*

10060

,.abscess-PE

Erythematous abscess mass noted superficially on _.
Measuring about _.
Punctate central exudative drainage.
Surrounding erythema.
Area is tender and warm to touch.
Fluctuance palpated.

,.abscess-loop-proc

Abscess I&D
Informed verbal consent was obtained.
Risks (including recurrence, unaesthetic scar, failure to resolve), benefits, and alternatives were reviewed with patient.
The area was prepared and draped in the usual sterile manner.
Local anesthetic with 1% lidlocaine w/ epinephrine instilled using 30G needle.
Abscess I&D'ed using No11 blade. Abscess was probed, and pus was drained.
Copious pus and caseous material removed.
Hemostats were introduced to break up loculations.
Cavity is irrigated with betadine.
A second incision, distal to the first one was made. A loop drain was passed through one incision, brought out through the other, and tied to itself.
Covered with a gauze.
Bleeding was minimal.
Pt tolerated procedure well.

,.abscess-proc

Abscess I&D
Informed verbal consent was obtained.
Risks (including recurrence, unaesthetic scar, failure to resolve), benefits, and alternatives were reviewed with patient.
The area was prepared and draped in the usual sterile manner.
Local anesthetic with 1% lidlocaine w/ epinephrine instilled using 30G needle.
Abscess I&D'ed using No11 blade. Abscess was probed, and pus was drained.
Copious pus and caseous material removed.
Cavity is irrigated with betadine.
Hemostats were introduced to break up loculations.
Sterile packing placed in the incision. Wound dressed with dry, sterile dressing.
Pt tolerated procedure well.
Bleeding was minimal.

,.anoscope-PE

Anoscopy revealed small internal hemorrhoid on right anterior segment.

,.anoscopy*

46600

,.debridement-wound-proc

Wound debridement
Location: _
Size: _ cm (_ sq cm)
Method of debridement:
Excisional - devitalized tissue was removed with a 10 blade scalpel.

Nonexcisional - irrigation with normal saline after using peroxide to clean blood.
Depth of debridement: skin and subcutaneous tissue (epidermis/dermis).
Debridement within wound margins.
Wound dressing applied.
Left to heal by secondary intention.

,.debridement-wound*<20sq-cm

97597

,.debridement-wound*ea-add20sq-cm

97598

,.dental-abscess

Pt c/o dental pain and swelling of gum.
Noted a pocket of fluid on gum.
No spontaneous drainage. no bleeding.
No fevers or chills.
Attempted to get dentist appointment but is unavailable until next week.

,.dental-abscess#

Dental abscess
S/p incision and drainage.
The patient tolerated the procedure well without complications.
Standard post-procedure care is explained and return precautions are given.
Rx antibiotic sent. amoxicillin-clavulanate - f/u dentist.
Return precautions discussed with patient, including excessive bleeding, fever, worsening of purulent discharge.

,.dental-abscess*

41800

,.dental-abscess-I&D-proc

Dental Abscess I&D
Right upper quadrant _periapical/ periodontal molar abscess
Informed verbal consent was obtained.
Risks (including recurrence, unaesthetic scar, failure to resolve), benefits, and alternatives were reviewed with patient.
The area was prepared in the usual, sterile manner.
Local anesthetic with 1% lidocaine w/ epinephrine instilled using 27ga needle.
Abscess I&D'ed using No11 blade. Abscess was probed, and purulent/ serosanguineous discharge was drained.
Abscess was probed, and pus was drained.
Bleeding was minimal.

,.dental-abscess-PE

Right upper quadrant _periapical/periodontal molar area.
Fluctuant mass palpated. Tender to touch.

,.diastasis-recti-PE

Diffuse fusiform bulge with valsalva maneuver, abdominal contents protrude into the thinned, bulged midline fascia.

,.excision#

_, right
Lesion excised today and sent to pathology.

Wound care instructions reviewed -- pt. to keep it dry for first 24 hours, then may shower starting tomorrow evening.
Advised to change bandaid and reapply triple antibiotic ointment daily.
F/u in 1 week for wound check and suture removal.

,.excisional-bx

Excisional biopsy
Elliptical excision of right _ lesion.
Measuring _ cm.
Skin was cleaned with 70% alcohol swab.
Area was anesthetized with 1% lidocaine.
Area was prepped in usual sterile fashion with 10% iodine swab and sterile drapes. Sterile gloves were used.
Elliptical excision performed on lesion with 15-blade.
Lesion removed in its entirety with scalpel and Adson forceps.
Hemostasis achieved.
 Intermediate repair: layered closure of subcutaneous tissue using 4-0 vicryl, _ sutures placed.
 Complex repair: undermining of the skin on both sides of the surgical wound was done to loosen the tissues and close the defect created.
Wound closed with 4-0 nylon suture, _ simple interrupted sutures placed.
Triple antibiotic ointment and bandaid applied.
Specimen sent to pathology

,.foreign-body-removal-proc

Location: right _
A foreign body embedded in subcutaneous tissue was identified.
Area was anesthetised using lidocaine 1%. A simple incision in the skin overlying the foreign body was made. The foreign body was retrieved using hemostats/forceps. The skin was not sutured allowing to heal secondarily.
Foreign body: _

„.foreign-body-removal-simple*

10120

„.global-sx-period*

99024

„.hemorrhoid-external#

Hemorrhoids, external
Dietary and lifestyle modification.
Fiber and fluids.
Sitz baths.
Po analgesics and topical anesthetics.
Desitin (zinc oxide topical).
Baby wipes.

„.hemorrhoids

Hemorrhoids
Pt c/o perianal pain/discomfort.
+ anal pruritus.
Endorses constipation.
No recent pregnancy.
+ spotting when wiping after BM.
Denies rectal bleeding.
Tender palpable rectal lesion.
Denies any rectal prolapsing mass.

„.hemorrhoids#

Hemorrhoids, internal
Dietary and lifestyle modification.

Fiber and fluids.
Short-term topical corticosteroids.
Grade 2-3 (prolapse/req manual reduction).
Consider rubber band ligation.

,.hernia#

Hernia, _
Symptomatic.
Candidate for surgical repair.
Warned about signs and symptoms of incarceration or obstruction.

,.hernia-PE

Reducible hernia palpated on _. Enlarges with valsalva maneuver.

,.hernia

Pt c/o discomfort and bulging mass on _.
Denies any pain.
No nausea, vomiting, constipation.

,.i&d-abscess*

10060

,.i&d-abscess-proc

Abscess I&D
Fluctuant area on right _.
Measuring _ cm.

Local anesthesia achieved with approx. 4 cc of 1% lidocaine without epinephrine. Area cleaned with 10% betadine solution.
3 mm incision made with sterile #11 blade scalpel. Copious amounts of yellow purulent discharge expressed. Sterile packing placed in the incision. Wound dressed with dry, sterile dressing. Pt tolerated procedure well.

,.i&d-boil-proc

Boil I&D
Location: right _.
Dimensions: 1x1 cm.
Consent obtained.
Local anesthesia achieved with ethyl chloride. Area cleaned with alcohol.
2 mm incision made with 18 G needle. Small amount of white thick material was expressed.
Hemostasis achieved with compression.
Wound dressed with dry, sterile dressing. Pt tolerated procedure well.

,.i&d-puncture-aspiration*abscess/cyst/boil/hematoma

10160

,.i&d-puncture-aspiration-proc-abscess/cyst/boil/hematoma

abscess/cyst/boil/hematoma puncture aspiration
Location: right _
Dimensions: 1x1 cm
Consent obtained.
Local anesthesia achieved with ethyl chloride. Area cleaned with alcohol.
Puncture aspiration made with 18 G needle. Small amount of white thick material was expressed.
Hemostasis achieved with compression.

Wound dressed with dry, sterile dressing. Pt tolerated procedure well.

,.laceration-proc

Laceration repair
Location: _
Size: _ cm

Patient was positioned appropriately. 5 cc lidocaine without epinephrine was used as a local anesthetic. NaCl was used for irrigation. Patient was sterile draped with wound exposed.
Wound closed with 4-0 nylon suture, _ simple interrupted sutures placed with good approximation. Procedure tolerated well without complications. Wound dressed with bacitracin and sterile gauze.

,.lipoma

Patient c/o a mass on _
Painless.
Increasing in size.
Present for several months.

,.lipoma#

Lipoma
Discussed treatment options.
Since lesion is bothersome and increasing in size.
Patient opted for excision.
Lesion sent for pathology.
Wound care discussed with patient.

,.lipoma-PE

4x4 cm superficial mass, mobile, not tender to palpation.

,.lipoma-excision

Lipoma excision
Location: right _
Measuring _ cm
Skin was cleaned with 70% alcohol swab.
Area was anesthetized with 1% lidocaine.
Area was prepped in usual sterile fashion with 10% iodine swab and sterile drapes. Sterile gloves were used.
Linear excision performed on lesion with 15-blade.
Lesion removed excised bluntly using small forceps and scissors.
Hemostasis achieved.
Intermediate repair: layered closure of subcutaneous tissue using 4-0 vicryl, _ sutures placed.
Wound closed with 4-0 nylon suture, _ simple interrupted sutures placed.
Triple antibiotic ointment and bandaid applied.
Specimen sent to pathology

,.pilonidal-abscess#

Pilonidal disease
With abscess.
I&D performed.
Healing by secondary intention.
Abx: Bactrim.
Analgesics.

,.pilonidal-ds

Pt c/o tailbone pain and swelling, worse when sitting.
Had some discharge.
Observed sinus tracts around the area.

,.pilonidal-ds#

Pilonidal disease
Asymptomatic.
Hair removal + local hygiene.

,.pilonidal-ds-PE

Sinus tract in the sacrococcygeal region, surrounding erythema, warmth, tenderness and fluctuance.

,.post-op-visit*

99024

,.sebaceous-cyst

Pt complains of cystic mass on _
Present for many months.
Increasing in size.
Some pain and tenderness.

,.sebaceous-cyst#

Sebaceous cyst
I&D/excision.
Wound care.

,.sebaceous-cyst-PE

Skin-colored subcutaneous nodule. _ cm. Mobile. Not tender to palpation.

,.sebaceous-cyst-i&d*

10060

,.sebaceous-cyst-i&d-proc

Sebaceous cyst I&D/excision
Location: right _
Dimensions: _ mm
Consent obtained.
Local anesthesia achieved with approx. 1 cc of 1% lidocaine with epinephrine. Area cleaned with 10% betadine solution.
3 mm incision made with sterile #11 blade scalpel. Small amount of white thick material was expressed.
Cyst wall was grasped with forceps and partially excised.
Hemostasis achieved with compression.
Wound dressed with dry, sterile dressing. Pt tolerated well.

,.sebaceous-cyst-proc

Sebaceous cyst excision
Location: right _
Size: _ cm
Preparation and technique: informed consent was obtained, position prone, sterile preparation of site (in usual fashion, with 10 % povidone iodine, draped to expose affected area, sterile gloves used), local anesthesia 1% lidocaine with epinephrine, 5 cc used.
Elliptical incision was made at center of lesion to include the punctum with 15-blade scalpel. Cyst wall gradually dissected away from the surrounding tissue carefully with Iris scissors and scalpel. Lesion removed in its entirety with scalpel and adson forceps, after cyst wall was freed from the surrounding tissue. While dissecting the lesion, small amount of white thick material was incidentally extruded from the punctum area, confirming diagnosis.
Hemostasis achieved.

Intermediate repair: layered closure of subcutaneous tissue using 4-0 vicryl, _ sutures placed.
Wound closed with 4-0 nylon suture, _ simple interrupted sutures placed.
Triple antibiotic ointment and bandaid applied.
Specimen sent to pathology

,.surgical-tray*

A4550

,.suture-removal

Here for suture removal.
Wound healing well.
Patient denies any bleeding or discharge.
No swelling or redness.
No fevers or chills.
Doing daily wound care.

,.suture-removal#

Wound healing well.
Continue wound care.

,.suture-removal-PE

Surgical wound clean and dry.

,.varicose-veins

Varicose-veins
C/o leg swelling and fatigue and aching with prolonged standing.

Reports skin changes.

,.varicose-veins#

Varicose veins
Sent for LE US.
Compression stockings.
Referred to vascular surgery for evaluation and possible phlebectomy.

,.varicose-veins-PE

Lower extremities dilated tortuous veins.

,.wound-debridement-1st20sqcm

11042

,.wound-debridement-subsq

11045

16.1 BILLING CODES

	EXCISION					
	trunk, arm, leg		scalp, neck, hand, feet, genitalia		face, ear, eyelid, nose, lip, muc.memb	
(cm)	B	M	B	M	B	M
<0.5	11400	11600	11420	11620	11440	11640
0.6-1	11401	11601	11421	11621	11441	11641
1.1-2	11402	11602	11422	11622	11442	11642
2.1-3	11403	11603	11423	11623	11443	11643
3.1-4	11404	11604	11424	11624	11444	11644
>4	11406	11606	11426	11626	11446	11646

B: Benign
M: Malignant

Excision of benign lesions includes simple repair of the wound. Intermediate or complex repairs are reported separately. See ,.repair-intermediate*, ,.repair-complex*.

For simple repair of lacerations, see ,.laceration* below.

For excision of malignant lesions 11600-11646, see ,.excision*mal-.

Intermediate or complex repairs of lacerations are reported separately. See ,.repair-intermediate*, ,.repair-complex*.

A wound repaired with glue or staples qualifies as a simple repair.

When multiple wounds are repaired, combine the lengths of those in the same classification and report them as a single item.

REPAIR								
	scalp, axillae, trunk, ext		trunk	neck, hands feet, genit	scalp, arm, leg	face, neck, hand, feet	Face, ear, eyelid, nose, lip, mm	
(cm)	S	I	C	I	C	C	S	(cm)
<2.5	12001	12031	13100	12041	13120	13131	12011	<2.5
2.6-7.5	12002	12032	13101	12042	13121	13132	12013	2.6-5
ea +5			13102		13122	13133	12014	5.1-7.5
7.6-12.5	12004	12034		12044			12015	7.6-12.5
12.6-20	12005	12035		12045			12016	12.6-20
20.1-30	12006	12036		12046			12017	20.1-30
30+	12007	12037		12047			12018	30+

S: Simple
I: Intermediate
C: Complex

SHAVING OF EPIDERMAL/DERMAL LESION			
(cm)	trunk, arm, leg	scalp, neck, hand	face
<0.5	11300	11305	11310
0.6-1	11301	11306	11311
1.1-2	11302	11307	11312
>2	11303	11308	11313

,.excision*trunk/arm/leg,<0.5cm

11400

,.excision*trunk/arm/leg,0.6-1cm

11401

,.excision*trunk/arm/leg,1-2cm

11402

,.excision*trunk/arm/leg,2-3cm

11403

,.excision*trunk/arm/leg,3-4cm

11404

,.excision*trunk/arm/leg,>4cm

11406

,.excision*scalp/neck/hand/ft<0.5cm

11420

,.excision*scalp/neck/hand/ft0.6-1cm
11421

,.excision*scalp/neck/hand/ft1-2cm
11422

,.excision*scalp/neck/hand/ft2-3cm
11423

,.excision*scalp/neck/hand/ft3-4cm
11424

,.excision*scalp/neck/hand/ft>4cm
11426

,.excision*face/ear<0.5cm
11440

,.excision*face/ear0.6-1cm
11441

,.excision*face/ear1-2cm

11442

,.excision*face/ear2-3cm

11443

,.excision*face/ear3-4cm

11444

,.excision*face/ear>4cm

11446

,.excision*mal-trunk/arm/leg,<0.5cm

11600

,.excision*mal-trunk/arm/leg,0.6-1cm

11601

,.excision*mal-trunk/arm/leg,1-2cm

11602

,.excision*mal-trunk/arm/leg,2-3cm
11603

,.excision*mal-trunk/arm/leg,3-4cm
11604

,.excision*mal-trunk/arm/leg,>4cm
11606

,.excision*mal-scalp/neck/hand/ft<0.5cm
11620

,.excision*mal-scalp/neck/hand/ft0.6-1cm
11621

,.excision*mal-scalp/neck/hand/ft1-2cm
11622

,.excision*mal-scalp/neck/hand/ft2-3cm
11623

,.excision*mal-scalp/neck/hand/ft3-4cm
11624

,.excision*mal-scalp/neck/hand/ft>4cm
11626

,.excision*mal-face/ear<0.5cm
11640

,.excision*mal-face/ear0.6-1cm
11641

,.excision*mal-face/ear1-2cm
11642

,.excision*mal-face/ear2-3cm
11643

,.excision*mal-face/ear3-4cm
11644

,.excision*mal-face/ear>4cm

11646

,.laceration*scalp,neck,axilla,gen,trunk,ext<2.5cm

12001

,.laceration*scalp,neck,axilla,gen,trunk,ext2.6-7.5cm

12002

,.laceration*scalp,neck,axilla,gen,trunk,ext7.6-12.5cm

12004

,.laceration*scalp,neck,axilla,gen,trunk,ext12.6-20cm

12005

,.laceration*scalp,neck,axilla,gen,trunk,ext20-30cm

12006

,.laceration*face,ears,eyelids,nose,lips<2.5cm

12011

,.laceration*face,ears,eyelids,nose,lips2.6-7.5cm

12012

,.repair-intermediate*scalp,axillae,trunk,ext<2.5cm

12031

,.repair-intermediate*scalp,axillae,trunk,ext2.6-7.5cm

12032

,.repair-intermediate*neck,hands/ft<2.5cm

12041

,.repair-intermediate*neck,hands/ft2.6-7.5cm

12042

,.repair-complex*trunk1-2.5cm

13100

,.repair-complex*trunk2.6-7.5cm

13101

,.repair-complex*scalp/arm/legs1-2.5cm

13120

,.repair-complex*scalp/arm/legs2.6-7.5cm

13121

,.repair-complex*face,neck,hand/ft1-2.5cm

13131

,.repair-complex*face,neck,hand/ft2.5-7.5cm

13132

17 URGENT CARE

,.abdominal-pain

C/o abdominal pain x days.
Location: generalized.
Constant.
Described as: cramps.
Worsens with food.
No fever, no chills.
No nausea, no vomiting.
Denies constipation.
LMP few wks ago. sexually active.
Denies vaginal discharge.
Denies vaginal bleeding.
Denies dysuria.

,.age-hpi

C/o abdominal pain, cramping, no diarrhea, watery, non-bloody diarrhea, multiple episodes.
C/o nausea, no vomiting, gastric content, non-bloody emesis, multiple episodes.
No fever or chills.

Symptoms present for days.
Decreased appetite, tolerating fluids.
No recent traveling, hospitalization, or use of antibiotics.
No new or street foods.
No sick contacts.

,.age#

Acute gastroenteritis
Likely viral. No labs or stool studies needed.
Not dehydrated or unable to maintain PO intake.
Reassured patient of self-limited course of disease.
Supportive care. Explained importance of rehydration.
Return if symptoms fail to improve or worsen.

,.asthma-exacerb#

Asthma exacerbation
Rx breathing tx and prednisone.

,.bite

C/o dog bite 1 day ago.
Location: hand while trying to separate a dog fight.
He is the dog owner. no abnormal behavior in animal.
Washed wound with soap and water.
Reports pain and swelling.
Denies any fevers or chills.

,.bite#

Bite, dog
Ppx abx with amoxicillin/clavulanate.
Tetanus vaccine given.

No need for rabies ig, will monitor pet for next 10 days.
Daily wound care.

,..centor-criteria

Mod. Centor criteria (<15/>44, fever, exudates, adenopathy, no cough) score:
  -1, 0, 1: No abx or throat cx needed. (risk of strep infx <10%)
  2, 3: rapid strep throat/cx, tx if + (risk of strep infx 15-32%)
  4, 5: tx empirically w/ abx (risk of strep infx 56%)

,..copd-exacerb#

\# COPD exacerbation
No need for oxygen. O2sat >90%
Bronchodilators/ICS
Short-course of prednisone.
Abx.

,..influenza

Pt c/o fever with cough.
C/o Headaches, myalgia, arthralgia.
Unvaccinated against influenza.
No rhinorrhea.
No sick contacts.

,..influenza#

\# Influenza
Tx w/ tamiflu.
Supportive care.

,.mva-hpi

MVA
Days ago.
Low velocity impact.
Rear impact.
No airbag deployed.
Pt was driver, was wearing a seatbelt.
No extrication.
Able to ambulate after accident.
No head trauma.
No LOC.

,.pharyngitis

C/o sore throat x days.
Endorses rhinorrhea, nasal congestion and cough, productive/dry.
+ fever.
No N/V, tolerating diet.

,.pharyngitis#

Pharyngitis
Likely viral. Centor score:
<2 - no rapid strep/cx necessary, no antibiotics indicated.
>= 4 treat empirically w/ antibiotics. Rx amoxicillin.
Supportive care.
Reassured NSAIDs should improve symptoms.
Tylenol prn fever.
Consider steroids.

,.pna#

Bacterial pneumonia
Empiric antibiotic.

Supportive care.

,.puncture-wound

Pt reports puncture injury with nail 1 day ago.
 Stepped on nail with footwear.
Object was clean.
No diabetes or chronic conditions.
Last tetanus immunization >10 yrs ago.

,.puncture-wound#

Puncture wound
Clean wound. Tetanus immunization.
No retained foreign objects. No need for imaging.
No evidence of deep infection.
Wound care.
Antibiotic prophylaxis for to provide coverage for S. aureus and beta-hemolytic streptococci with cephalexin.
Additional coverage for plantar puncture wounds with levofloxacin.

,.subungual-hematoma

Pt reports injury to toenail days ago.
Noted darkening of nail bed.
C/o significant discomfort with pressure.

,.subungual-hematoma#

Subungual hematoma
Painful. Trephination done to relieve compression.
Sent pt for X-ray to r/o fracture.
Wound care. Pain control.

,.subungual-hematoma*

11740

,.subungual-hematoma-PE

Blue-black discoloration of the nail plate due to the accumulation of blood beneath the nail plate.

,.subungual-hematoma-trephination

Subungual hematoma trephination
Consent obtained from patient. Discussed risks and benefits.
No digital block was necessary.
Nail cleaned with povidone iodine.
Using a movie high-temp cautery the tip of the device was pressed against the nail in the center making a 3 mm hole. Blood drained. Puncture site was then covered with a sterile gauze.
Patient tolerated procedure well.

,.uri#

URI
Likely viral.
Reassurance. Supportive care.
Increase fluid intake, rest.
Fever control with Tylenol/Ibuprofen.
OTC decongestant. pseudoephedrine, Benadryl.
Salt water gargles, ice chips to soothe throat tid. Lozenges.
Increase humidity using humidifier by bedside. Exposure to steam for expectoration.
Nasal saline prn.
Return to clinic if not improved over the next several days, or if getting worse.

,.uri-adult

Presents with rhinorrhea, nasal congestion, headache, sore throat, cough, non-productive.
Symptoms present for days.
No SOB/wheezing.
No fever.
No sick contacts.

,.uri-adults-PE

General: No acute distress. Awake and conversant.
Eyes: Normal conjunctiva, anicteric. Round symmetric pupils.
ENT: Tympanic membranes are clear, No sinus tenderness, Mild pharyngeal erythema, no exudates, Nasal mucosa erythematous and edematous. Clear rhinorrhea.
Neck: Neck is supple. Tender anterior lymphadenopathy.
Respiratory: Respirations are non-labored. Lungs are clear to auscultation. No wheezing.
Skin: Warm. No rashes or ulcers.
Psych: Alert and oriented. Cooperative, Appropriate mood and affect, Normal judgment.
CV: Normal rate, Regular rhythm, No murmur.
MSK: Normal ambulation. No clubbing or cyanosis.
Neuro: Sensation and CN II-XII grossly normal.

,.uri-pediatric

Presents with rhinorrhea for days.
No fever.
Using tylenol/ibuprofen.
Pulling at ears.
Associated cough. Non-productive, clear sputum.
Fussy and clingy.
Decreased appetite; taking fluids well.
>3 wet diapers in the last 24 hrs.

No vomiting.
No diarrhea.
Positive sick contacts at home/daycare.
Immunizations up to date.

,.uri-pediatric#

Upper Respiratory Infection
Likely viral. No respiratory distress. Tolerating fluids.
Reassurance. Supportive care.
Increase fluid intake.
Fever control with Tylenol/Ibuprofen. Dosage per weight.
Increase humidity using humidifier by bedside or exposure to steam from a shower.
Saline drops and bulb suctioning prn.
Return to clinic if not improved over the next several days, or if getting worse.
Return precautions discussed w/ parents (fever 100.4, inc respiratory distress, not tolerating fluids or decrease urine output).

,.uri-peds-PE

General: No acute distress. Well nourished and developed.
Eye: Normal conjunctiva, anicteric.
HENT: Tympanic membranes are clear, No sinus tenderness, Mild pharyngeal erythema, no exudates, Nasal mucosa erythematous and edematous. Clear rhinorrhea.
Neck: Supple, no tender anterior lymphadenopathy.
Respiratory: Respirations are non-labored. Lungs are clear to auscultation.
Skin: Warm. No rashes or ulcers.
Psych: Awake and alert. Cooperative.
Cardiovascular: Normal rate, Regular rhythm, No murmur.
Gastrointestinal: Soft, Non-tender, Non-distended.
MSK: Moves all extremities. No cyanosis.

,.uti-hpi

Pt c/o dysuria, urinary frequency and urgency for days.
No fever, chills.
No flank pain. No N/V.
No hematuria.
No suprapubic pain.
No malodorous urine.
Denies vaginal d/c.
No recent UTI or abx use.

,.uti#

\# UTI, uncomplicated
Urine dipstick: + LE, + Nitrates.
Start empiric abx.
Nitrofurantoin 100 mg bid X 5 days
 Trimethoprim-sulfamethoxazole 160/800 mg bid x 3 days.
Consider cranberry juice.
Return prn failure to improve.

,.uti#complicated

\# UTI, complicated
Mild/mod severity. Outpatient management.
Urine dipstick: + LE, + Nitrates.
Start empiric abx.
IM ceftriaxone given.
Trimethoprim-sulfamethoxazole 160/800 mg bid x 7 days.
Sent for urinalysis and urine culture.
F/u susceptibility.
Consider cranberry juice.
Return prn failure to improve.

,.uti-PE

General: No acute distress. Awake and conversant.
Eyes: Normal conjunctiva, anicteric. Round symmetric pupils.
ENT: Hearing grossly intact. No nasal discharge.
Neck: Neck is supple. No masses or thyromegaly.
Respiratory: Respirations are non-labored. No wheezing.
Abdomen: soft, mild suprapubic tenderness.
Back: no CVA tenderness.
Skin: Warm. No rashes or ulcers.
Psych: Alert and oriented. Cooperative, Appropriate mood and affect, Normal judgment.
CV: No lower extremity edema.
MSK: Normal ambulation. No clubbing or cyanosis.
Neuro: Sensation and CN II-XII grossly normal.

18 INPATIENT/SNF

,..acs#inpt

\# Acute coronary syndrome
 Neg troponin - unstable angina
+ Tp - NSTEMI
MONA.
ACEI, BB, statins.
PCI.
Admit to telemetry. Continue heparin gtt.
Appreciate cardiology consultation and recommendations.

,..afib-rvr#inpt

\# Afib w/ RVR
Hemodynamically stable.
Admit to ICU for rate control with diltiazem gtt.
Continue anticoagulation.

,..alcohol-withdrawal#inpt

\# Alcohol withdrawal

Admit to ICU for CIWA protocol.
Mechanical restraints as needed.
Volume resuscitation/banana bag.
Replete K, Mg, PO4.

,.asthma-exacerb#inpt

Asthma exacerbation
Admit for breathing treatments and IV steroids.
Continue oxygen supplementation.

,.chf-exacerb#inpt

CHF exacerbation
CXR w/ plum edema, pleural effusions, cardiomegaly.
Elevated BNP.
Precipitants: _
Admit to telemetry.
IV diuretics with Lasix.
Prn venodilators with morphine and nitrates.
Oxygen supplementation per protocol.
Elevate head of bed.

,.copd-exacerb#inpt

COPD exacerbation
Admit for breathing treatments, IV steroids and antibiotics.
Continue oxygen supplementation.

,.cp#inpt

Chest pain
MONA, supportive care.
Admit to telemetry r/o ACS.

Hemodynamically stable.
EKG w/o evidence of acute ischemia.
Negative troponin. Trend.
Stress test ordered.

,..cva#inpt

\# Stroke
Head CT unremarkable.
No tPA given.
Admit to telemetry. Permissive HTN.
Started asa and statin.
W/u to assess etiology:
MRI. MR angio head & neck.
2d echo, carotid US.

,..cva-tpa#inpt

\# Stroke
Head CT unremarkable.
tPA given.
Admit to ICU.
BP <180/105.
Hold asa x24 hrs.
Started statin.
W/u to assess etiology:
MRI. MR angio head & neck.
2d echo, carotid US.

,..death-note

Called by nursing to see patient regarding unresponsiveness. Patient was found to be breathless, pulseless, and without heart sounds, blood pressure, and corneal reflexes. The patient was pronounced dead at 4:25 AM on June

18, 2017. Daughter at bedside. Refused both anatomic gifts and autopsy. The funeral home will be contacted.

,.diverticulitis#inpt

Diverticulitis
First episode.
No abscess or perforation.
No signs of acute abdomen or sepsis.
Admit for pain control, NPO, IVF, NGT.
IV abs for GNR and anaerobic coverage.

,.dka#inpt

DKA
Admit to ICU for insulin gtt. Aggressive IV fluids.
No evidence of infection or other precipitants.
Monitor anion gap.
Pseudohyponatremia - monitor.
Electrolyte repletion. K<4.5
HCO3, pH>7
PO4 >1

,.dm-foot-ulcer#inpt

Diabetic foot ulcer
Limb-threatening/systemic toxicity.
IV abx (vanco/zosyn). f/u cultures.
No evidence of osteomyelitis on imaging.
Elevation, wound care.
Appreciate podiatry evaluation and consultation for possible surgical debridement.

,.gi-bleed#inpt

\# GI bleeding
Hemodynamically stable.
Admit to ICU.
Continue PPI ggt, Octreotide gtt. Ceftriaxone x5d.
Monitor anemia.
NPO. Continue IV fluids.
Hold anticoagulants/reverse coagulopathy:
 Keep plts >50k
 FFP & vit K to normalize PT/INR <1.5
Appreciate GI consult and recommendations.
Consider endoscopy.

,.hhs#inpt

\# Hyperosmolar hyperglycemic state
Admit to ICU for insulin gtt. Aggressive IV fluids (NS->1/2NS).
No evidence of infection or other precipitants.
No ketoacidosis. Serum osmolality >320.
Monitor renal function.

,.htn-emerg#inpt

\# Hypertensive emergency
With evidence of end-organ damage.
Monitor renal fx.
Admit for gradual BP lowering.
Continue Nicardipine gtt.
No acute CHF. Normal UDS.

,.inpt-subjective

Afebrile.
On IV antibiotics.

No complaints or overnight events otherwise.

,..nstemi#inpt

Acute coronary syndrome
 Neg troponin - unstable angina
+ Tp - NSTEMI
MONA.
ACEI, BB, statins.
PCI.
Admit to telemetry. Continue heparin gtt.
Appreciate cardiology consultation and recommendations.

,..pancreatitis#inpt

Pancreatitis
Admit for pain control.
IV fluid resuscitation.
NPO. Early enteral feeding.
No evidence of gallstones.
No evidence of pancreatic necrosis on imaging.
F/u lipid panel r/o hypertriglyceridemia.

,..pe-adult-ICU

General: No acute distress. Sedated and intubated.
Eyes: Normal conjunctiva, anicteric. Round symmetric pupils.
ENT: Oral mucosa is moist. OG tube in place.
Neck: Neck is supple. No masses or thyromegaly. No jugular venous distention.
Respiratory: Intubated. Lungs are clear to auscultation.
Abdomen: soft, nontender, nondistended, no guarding or rebound.
Skin: Warm. No rashes or ulcers.
CV: Normal heart sounds, no murmurs. No lower extremity edema.
MSK: No obvious deformities. No clubbing or cyanosis.

Neuro: Patient is sedated.

,.pe-adult-inpt

General: No acute distress. Awake and conversant.
Eyes: Normal conjunctiva, anicteric. Round symmetric pupils.
ENT: Hearing grossly intact. No nasal discharge. Oral mucosa is moist.
Neck: Neck is supple. No masses or thyromegaly.
Respiratory: Respirations are non-labored. Lungs are clear to auscultation.
Abdomen: soft, nontender, nondistended, no guarding or rebound.
Skin: Warm. No rashes or ulcers.
Psych: Alert and oriented. Cooperative, Appropriate mood and affect, Normal judgment.
CV: Normal heart sounds, no murmurs. No lower extremity edema.
MSK: No obvious deformities. No clubbing or cyanosis.
Neuro: Sensation and CN II-XII grossly normal.

,.pna#inpt

Bacterial pneumonia
No sepsis. Hemodynamically stable.
No respiratory failure.
Admit for supportive care.
IV antibiotics.
Oxygen supplementation.
f/u cultures, urinary Ag.

,.sbo#inpt

Small bowel obstruction
Admit for IVF, GI decompression with NGT.
Supportive care, bowel rest, NPO.
Correction of metabolic abnormalities.
No signs of bowel compromise.

".sepsis-reeval

Sepsis Re-evaluation: Vital signs, cardiopulmonary, capillary refill, pulses and skin findings were reviewed and assessed. The focused exam and data suggests [adequate] fluid resuscitation.

".sepsis#inpt

Sepsis
Severe - w/ organ dysfunction, hypotension, lactic acidosis, oliguria, change MS.
Admit to telemetry for aggressive IV hydration.
Continue empiric IV abx.
f/u cultures.
Early goal-directed therapy:
Target MAP >65
UOP > 0.5 mL/kg/h
Lactate clearance > 20%/2h

".septic-shock#inpt

Septic shock
w/ hypotension not responding to fluid resuscitation.
Admit to ICU for aggressive IV hydration and vasopressors.
Continue empiric IV abx.
f/u cultures.
Steroids?
Early goal-directed therapy:
Target MAP >65
UOP > 0.5 mL/kg/h
Lactate clearance > 20%/2h

".snf-cc

SNF admission to _
Date of admission: _

,.soft-tissue-infx#inpt

Soft tissue infection
Cellulitis/ No abscess.
Meets sepsis criteria. Not immunosuppressed.
Start Vancomycin for beta-hemolytic Streptococcus and MRSA coverage.
De-escalate antibiotic therapy once pathogen and susceptibilities are known and clinical response.
Supportive care. Extremity elevation.

,.stemi#inpt

STEMI
s/p PCI.
Admit to ICU.
Loading doses of Brillinta and heparin given.
ACEI, BB, statins.
asa, oxygen per protocol.
2d echo.
Appreciate cardiology consultation and recommendations.

,.syncope#inpt

Syncope
Unexplained etiology. possibly vasovagal.
Reflex/neurocardiogenic syncope 2/2 _.
Check orthostatic vital signs.
No suspicion for cardiac etiology. normal EKG, no hx of cardiac ds.
Admit to telemetry for observation.
2d echocardiogram ordered.
No suspicion for neurologic etiology, including seizures or CVA. no head trauma. CT head negative.
Normal CBC and BMP w/o evidence of anemia or electrolyte abnormalities.

18.1 BILLING CODES

	hospital care (admit)	observation care (obs)	nursing facility care (snf)
Initial (h&p)	99221	99218	99304
	99222	99219	99305
	99223	99220	99306
Subsequent (f/u)	99231	99224	99307
	99232	99225	99308
	99233	99226	99309
			99310
Discharge (d/c)	99238	99217	99315
>30 min	99239		99316
		annual snf assessment	99318

	inpatient	ED
Consult*	99251	99281
	99252	99282
	99253	99283
	99254	99284
	99255	99285

	1st 30-74 min	add 30 min
Critical care	99291	99292
ALS	99288	

	Prolonged services hospital or SNF	
	face-to-face	no direct contact
1st hour	99356	99358
add 30 min	99357	99359

* *consult f/u = subsequent hospital care (admit-f/u). Medicare doesn't accept consult codes - use hospital care EM codes*

,.em-inpt-admit-h&p-1

99221

,.em-inpt-admit-h&p-2

99222

,.em-inpt-admit-h&p-3

99223

,.em-inpt-admit-f/u-1

99231

,.em-inpt-admit-f/u-2

99232

,.em-inpt-admit-f/u-3
99233

,.em-inpt-admit-d/c-1
99238

,.em-inpt-admit-d/c-2
99239

,.em-inpt-obs-h&p-1
99218

,.em-inpt-obs-h&p-2
99219

,.em-inpt-obs-h&p-3
99220

,.em-inpt-obs-f/u-1
99224

,.em-inpt-obs-f/u-2
99225

,.em-inpt-obs-f/u-3

99226

,.em-inpt-obs-d/c

99217

,.em-inpt-consult-1

99251

,.em-inpt-consult-2

99252

,.em-inpt-consult-3

99253

,.em-inpt-consult-4

99254

,.em-inpt-consult-5

99255

,.em-inpt-consult-ed-1

99281

,.em-inpt-consult-ed-2
99282

,.em-inpt-consult-ed-3
99283

,.em-inpt-consult-ed-4
99284

,.em-inpt-consult-ed-5
99285

,.em-inpt-critical-30-74
99291

,.em-inpt-critical+30
99292

,.em-inpt-critical-als
99288

,.em-inpt-prolong-60
99356

,.em-inpt-prolong+30
99357

,.em-inpt-prolong-indirect-60
99358

,.em-inpt-prolong-indirect+30
99359

,.em-snf-h&p-1
99304

,.em-snf-h&p-2
99305

,.em-snf-h&p-3
99306

,.em-snf-f/u-1
99307

,.em-snf-f/u-2
99308

,..em-snf-f/u-3
99309

,..em-snf-f/u-4
99310

,..em-snf-d/c-1
99315

,..em-snf-d/c-2
99316

,..em-snf-annual
99318

,..em-snf-prolong-60
99356

,..em-snf-prolong+30
99357

,..em-snf-prolong-indirect-60
99358

,.em-snf-prolong-indirect+30
99359

,.time-inpt-d/c
Time spent on discharge, coordinating care with RN staff and/or consultant, examining patient, discussing findings and plans with patient and/or family, documentation, coding is greater than 30 minutes; greater than 50% time on coordinating care and counseling patient and/or family.

19 MESSAGES: LAB, IMAGING, PATH RESULTS

,.aaa+EN

There was a small aneurysm on your aorta.
We will closely monitor and repeat the ultrasound in one year.
No treatment needed for now.

,.aaa+SP

Hay un pequeño aneurisma en su aorta.
Vamos a monitorear. Por ahora no es necesario ningún tratamiento.
Repetiremos el ultrasonido en un año.

,.aaa-EN

Your ultrasound study showed no evidence of abdominal aortic aneurysm (AAA). This was a screening test and no further studies are needed.

,.aaa-SP

Su estudio de ultrasonido no demostró evidencia de aneurisma aórtico abdominal. Este estudio es de detección y no necesita estudios adicionales.

,.carotid-us-EN

Your ultrasound showed <50% obstruction of the carotid arteries. There is currently no need for any further evaluation or procedures. Unless you develop any symptoms we can repeat the ultrasound in three years.

,.carotid-us-SP

Su ultrasonido mostró <50% de obstrucción de sus arterias carótidas. No es necesario ningún procedimiento por ahora.
Si no tiene ningún síntoma el ultrasonido debe repetirse en tres años.

,.colon-notdone-EN

Your colon cancer screening test was not performed due to improper collection of the stool sample. Please repeat tests.

,.colon-notdone-SP

Su examen de detección temprana de colon de cáncer no fue realizado debido a que el espécimen de popó no fue correctamente proporcionado. Por favor repita el estudio.

,.colon-screen-EN

Your colon cancer screen was negative. Continue with your yearly routine screening.

,.colon-screen-SP

Su prueba de detección de cáncer de colon fue normal. Esta prueba es recomendada una vez al año.

,.ct-lung-EN

Your imaging test revealed small lung nodules that appeared benign. Continued yearly screening is recommended until age 77, or until you stop smoking for 15 years.

,.ct-lung-SP

Su estudio de imagen mostró pequeños nódulos en sus pulmones que parecen benignos. Se recomienda repetir el estudio cada año hasta que cumpla 77 años o hasta que deje de fumar por 15 años.

,.inr-EN

Your INR is at goal. Continue same dose of warfarin. Recheck INR in one month.

,.inr-SP

Su INR esta bien. Continue la misma dosis de warfarina. Cheque su INR en un mes.

„.lab-cholesterol-EN-no-med

Your cholesterol is high. No medications are needed at this point. Improve your diet and increase your physical activity. We will monitor your cholesterol levels in the future.

„.lab-cholesterol-SP-no med

Su colesterol está alto. No es necesario empezar medicamento por ahora, pero necesita hacer más ejercicio y mejorar su dieta. Estaremos monitoreando su colesterol en el futuro.

„.lab-cholesterol-high-EN

Your cholesterol level is high. Your 10-year calculated risk for having a heart attack or a stroke is 15%. The American Heart Association recommends starting a cholesterol lowering medicine called statin for adults 40 to 75 years of age with a risk >7.5%. We will discuss starting the medication during your next visit. I also recommend a heart healthy diet and to increase your physical activity. Call my office if you have any questions. Otherwise continue with all your meds and a healthy lifestyle.

„.lab-cholesterol-high-SP

Su colesterol está elevado. Su riesgo calculado de tener un ataque al corazón o embolia en los siguientes 10 años es de 13.6%. La Asociación Americana del Corazón recomienda empezar una medicina para reducir el colesterol llamada estatina para adultos de 40 a 75 años con un riesgo >7.5%. Discutiremos empezar el medicamento durante su siguiente visita. También le recomiendo una dieta sana e incrementar su actividad física. Llame a mi oficina si tiene alguna pregunta. De lo contrario continúe con el resto de sus medicamentos y un estilo de vida saludable.

,.lab-cholesterol-stable-EN

Your cholesterol is well controlled. No medication changes are needed at this point. Continue with a healthy diet and physical activity. We will monitor your cholesterol levels in the future.

,.lab-cholesterol-stable-SP

Su colesterol está bien controlado. No es necesario cambiar sus medicamentos. Continúe con una dieta sana y ejercicio. Estaremos monitoreando sus niveles de colesterol en el futuro.

,.lab-dm-ctrl-EN

Your diabetes is well controlled.

,.lab-dm-ctrl-SP

Su diabetes está bien controlada.

,.lab-hepatitis-EN

Your hepatitis screening test was negative.

,.lab-hepatitis-SP

Su resultado de hepatitis fue negativo.

,.lab-measles-EN

You have immunity against measles.

,.lab-measles-SP

El laboratorio muestra que tiene inmunidad contra el sarampión.

,.lab-microalbuminuria-EN

Your kidneys are "spilling a little protein" (microalbuminuria).
No medications are needed at this point.
We will monitor your microalbumin levels in the future.

,.lab-microalbuminuria-SP

Sus riñones están "tirando un poco de proteína" (microalbuminuria).
No necesita nuevos medicamentos.
Vamos a monitorear sus niveles de microalbúmina en el futuro.

,.lab-nl-EN

All your lab results are normal. Continue with all your medications and a healthy lifestyle.

,.lab-nl-SP

Todos los resultados de laboratorio son normales. Continúe con sus medicamentos y un estilo de vida saludable.

,.lab-nl-rest-EN

The rest of your lab results are normal. Continue with current medical management and a healthy lifestyle.

,.lab-nl-rest-SP

El resto de los resultados de laboratorio son normales. Continúe el actual manejo médico y un estilo de vida saludable.

,.lab-prediabetes-EN

Your lab result is in the prediabetic range. No need for medications for now. We will repeat the lab in the future. continue with a healthy diet and active lifestyle.

,.lab-prediabetes-SP

Sus resultados de laboratorio muestran que su azúcar está en el rango de prediabetes. No es necesario empezar ningún medicamento pero necesita hacer más ejercicio y mejorar su dieta. Estaremos monitoreando los laboratorios.

,.lab-testosterone-low-EN

Your testosterone was low. Further testing is needed. We will recheck you testosterone level as well as other hormones like LH/FSH. Please make sure you do the test before 10 AM to get an accurate level.

,.lab-testosterone-low-SP

Su nivel de testosterona está bajo. Se necesitan más estudios. Vamos a checar otra vez su nivel de testosterona y otras hormonas (LH/FSH). Asegúrese de hacer la prueba antes de las 10 AM para obtener un resultado certero.

,.lab-testosterone-rep-SP

Su testosterona salió baja otra vez. Los niveles de FSH y LH están altos. Esto significa que sus testículos están produciendo menos testosterona y no es un problema metabólico. Si todavía tiene síntomas como depresión, menos apetito sexual o vigor podemos considerar empezar tratamiento con testosterona. Tiene que estar consciente de los posibles efectos secundarios incluyendo el aumento de su riesgo de eventos cardiovasculares como embolias o ataques al corazón, cáncer y crecimiento de la próstata, colesterol alto, entre otros. Si decide empezar el tratamiento necesitamos otros laboratorios para saber su nivel de PSA, enzimas del hígado, colesterol, y descartar anemia. También necesita un examen de próstata. Por favor haga una cita si desea empezar el tratamiento.

,.lab-testosterone-rep-EN

Your testosterone was low again. Further testing shows that your FSH and LH were high. Which means your testicles are producing less testosterone and it is not a metabolic problem. If you are still feeling symptomatic (decreased vigor, libido, depression) we can consider treatment with testosterone. You have to be aware of the potential side effects including increasing your risk of cardiovascular events, prostate hypertrophy/cancer, high cholesterol, among others. If you decide to start treatment we need some baseline lab test to check your PSA, liver, cholesterol and evaluate for anemia. You will also need a prostate exam. Please schedule an appointment if you wish to start treatment.

,.lab-thyroid-EN

Your thyroid lab was mildly out of range. There is no need for a medication but contact us if your fatigue symptoms persist.

,.lab-thyroid-SP

El resultado de la tiroides salió un poco fuera de lo normal. No es necesario empezar un medicamento pero contáctenos si persisten los síntomas de cansancio.

,.lab-vasectomy-EN

The sperm count test suggests that your vasectomy was a success. The lab shows no sperm at all. You can discontinue using other contraceptive methods.

,.lab-vasectomy-SP

La prueba de esperma sugiere que su vasectomía fue realizada con éxito. El laboratorio no mostró ningún espermatozoide. Puede dejar de usar otros métodos anticonceptivos.

,.lab-vasectomy-rep-EN

The lab test showed some sperm. Please repeat the test in one month. Ideally you should have 15-20 ejaculations after your vasectomy. Continue using other birth control methods in the meantime.

,.lab-vasectomy-rep-SP

El laboratorio mostró algunos espermatozoides. Por favor repita la prueba en un mes. Lo ideal es tener de 15-20 eyaculaciones después de la vasectomía. Continue usando otros métodos anticonceptivos.

,.lung-ca-screen-EN

Your lung cancer screening did not show evidence of lung cancer. Routine follow up in one year is recommended.

,.lung-ca-screen-SP

Su prueba de detección de cáncer de pulmón fue normal. Esta prueba es recomendada una vez al año.

,.mammo-nl-EN

Your mammogram did not show evidence of breast cancer. Routine follow up is recommended.

,.mammo-nl-SP

Su mamograma no mostró evidencia de cáncer de seno. Continúe con su mamograma cada dos años.

,.pap-nl-EN

Your pap smear was normal. Routine follow up is recommended. Your next pap smear should be done in 5 years.

,.pap-nl-SP

Su papanicolaou fue normal. Su siguiente papanicolaou debe hacerlo dentro de 5 años.

,.path-EN

Your pathology result was benign.

,.path-SP

Su resultado de patología salió normal.

,.path-vasectomy-EN

The pathology result shows that the procedure was done correctly. Do not forget to bring your semen analysis to the lab in two months.

,.path-vasectomy-SP

Su resultado de patología mostró que la vasectomía fue realizada correctamente, removiendo una porción de los conductos deferentes. No olvide traer su estudio de semen al laboratorio en dos meses.

,.prostate-psa-lab-EN

Your serum prostatic antigen (PSA) is normal. This is usually elevated when there is prostate cancer. Currently there is no consensus regarding prostate cancer screening. If you desire we can repeat your test in 2 to 4 years.

,.prostate-psa-lab-SP

Su nivel de antígeno prostático (PSA) está normal. Los niveles de PSA generalmente aumenta cuando hay cáncer de próstata. Actualmente no hay un consenso en cuanto a recomendaciones para detectar cáncer de próstata. Si lo desea podemos repetir la prueba en 2 a 4 años.

,.strike

You have signed a Controlled Substance Agreement for your prescription of _.

You are being issued a strike today for: _ Non consistent urine drug test. Prescribed drug was not present in your urine.

A strike means you have violated your Controlled Substance Agreement. We take very seriously in view of the risks of opioids as well as the National Opioid Epidemic.

Any additional strikes may cause us to stop prescribing opiates altogether for you. You may be required to see another specialist, obtain other non-opioid treatments and change your medication and/or dosage. If there are further violations or strikes, we may also consider discharge from the practice.

Please return this letter signed prior to next medication refill.

I understand this and agreed to no further violations:

Signature: _____

Date: _____

,.strike-letterx2

You have signed a Controlled Substance Agreement for your prescription of hydrocodone, tramadol, and clonazepam.

You are being issued a strike today for: Non consistent urine drug test. Methamphetamines present in your urine.

A strike means you have violated your Controlled Substance Agreement. We take very seriously in view of the risks of opioids as well as the National Opioid Epidemic.

This is your second strike. This recurrent violation to our contract means we will stop prescribing opiates altogether for you. To continue with your treatment you are required to see another specialist, obtain other non-opioid treatments and/or change your medication to a non opioid or benzodiazepine. You are welcome to continue in our practice to address all you other medical problems not related to conditions for which you take these medications.

Please return this letter signed in order to get a 30 day supply of your medications to give you a chance to find a different provider outside our clinic.

I understand this and agreed to no longer get control substances from this clinic:

Signature: _____

Date: _____

,.uds

Pt needs UDS prior to next refill. Needs to go to lab every 4 months.

,.urine-cx+EN

The urine culture confirmed a urinary tract infection.
Please finish your antibiotic.
Return to clinic if your symptoms do not improve.

,.urine-cx+SP

El cultivo de orina confirmó su infección urinaria.
Por favor termine de tomar el antibiótico.

Regrese a la clínica si sus síntomas no mejoran.

,.us-nl-EN

Your ultrasound was normal.

,.us-nl-SP

Su ultrasonido salió normal.

,.xray-knee-EN

Your xray showed knee osteoarthritis.

,.xray-knee-SP

Su radiografía mostró artritis de su rodilla.

,.xray-nl-EN

Your xray was normal.

,.xray-nl-SP

Su radiografía salió normal.

20 MISCELLANEOUS

,.abx

Delayed antibiotic prescription if condition persist or worsens - fever.

,.b12

Patient does not have a documented vitamin B12 deficiency however she reports improvement of symptoms with B12 injections. Probably a placebo effect.
IM vit b12 inj given in clinic.

,.barbiturates

Your urine drug screen came back positive for barbiturates (butalbital). This could be a false-positive from chronic use of NSAIDs like ibuprofen or naproxen. However, if you are taking butalbital or any other barbiturates please disclose this during your next visit so that we can amend your controlled substance agreement. These medications are commonly used for migraine headaches and can produce sedation. Brand names include Fioricet, Esgic, Orbivan.

,.cpo-home-health

Care Plan Oversight

Patient was started on home health on 1/1/19 under my supervision.
Charts, reports and treatment plans were reviewed.
At least 15 minutes were spent on care plan oversight and/or care coordination during this calendar month.

,.cpo-home-health*15

99374

,.cpo-home-health*30

99375

,.cpo-hospice

Care Plan Oversight

Patient was admitted to hospice on 3/26/18 under my supervision.
Charts, reports and treatment plans were reviewed.
At least 15 minutes were spent on care plan oversight and/or care coordination during this calendar month.

,.cpo-hospice*15

99377

,.cpo-hospice*30

99378

,.diabetic-shoes

Diabetic Statement
Statement of Certifying Physician for Therapeutic Shoes

I certify that this patient has diabetes mellitus.

I certify that this patient has one or more of the following conditions:
_ history of partial or complete amputation of the foot.
_ history of previous foot ulceration.
_ history of pre-ulcerative callus.
_ peripheral neuropathy with evidence of callus formation.
_ foot deformity.
_ poor circulation.

I am treating this patient under a comprehensive plan of care for his/her diabetes.

This patient needs special shoes (depth or custom-molded shoes) because of his/her diabetes.

Date last seen for diabetic exam: _

,.disability

I filled out disability paperwork to the best of my knowledge.
Pt declined functional capacity evaluation testing due to cost.

,.f2f-cane

Face to Face Encounter Documentation

I certify that this patient is or has been under my care and that I had a face-to-face encounter that meets the physician face-to-face encounter requirements with this patient within the last six months. The major reason for the visit was a mobility examination.

My clinical findings support the need for a cane because:
The patient has a mobility limitation that significantly impairs his/her ability to participate in one or more mobility-related activities of daily living (MRADL).
Medical condition: _

Patient can safely use a cane and it will sufficiently resolve the ability to perform the above activities.

,.f2f-home-health

Home Health Certification/Documentation of Face-to-Face Encounter
Patient: _
DOB: _

Home Health Certification
I certify that, based on my findings, the following services are medically necessary home health services and initiate the orders for these services:

_Skilled Nursing
_Physical Therapy
_Speech Therapy
_Occupational Therapy

To provide the following care/treatments:

_Skilled Nursing: Observation and assessment of medical condition, Patient-Caregiver education of a Disease Process, Medication Education and Management, Direct care for Wound/Ostomy Care, Cardiac care, Diabetes care, Pain Management, Infusion, Injections, Catheter Care.
_Physical Therapy: Transfer and Mobility training, Therapeutic exercises, manual therapy, assistive devices, ADL training and adaptive equipment, neuromuscular retraining, perceptual/cognitive training, home safety evaluation, home exercise program.

_Speech Therapy: Swallow safety.

I certify that this patient is confined to his/her home and needs intermittent services as shown above. This patient is or has been under my care, and I have authorized the services on this certification. If this patient is no longer under my care, the care has been handed off to another physician and is so documented within our records.

Face to Face Encounter Documentation
I certify that this patient is or has been under my care and that I, or a nurse practitioner or physician's assistant working with me, had a face-to-face encounter that meets the physician face-to-face encounter requirements with this patient on:

Face-to-Face Encounter Date _4/11/19

The encounter with the patient was in whole, or in part, for the following medical condition, which is the primary reason for home health care.

Medical Condition: _Stroke

My clinical findings support the need for the above services because:

_The patient or caregiver's knowledge deficit. The patient is medically labile, complex, or on a high risk medical regime, at high risk for rehospitalization, unable to provide self-care, with functional impairment, necessary for the treatment of the illness or injury.

Further, I certify that my clinical findings support that this patient is homebound (i.e. absences from home require considerable and taxing effort and are for medical reasons or religious services or infrequently or of short duration when for other reasons) because:

_The Patient is unable to leave home due to illness or injury, requires the assistance of a device, other person, or special transportation, leaving home requires considerable and taxing effort and are restricted to medical reasons or of short duration.

Physician: _

Date: _

,.f2f-hospital-bed

Face to Face Encounter Documentation

I certify that this patient is or has been under my care and that I had a face-to-face encounter that meets the physician face-to-face encounter requirements with this patient within the last six months. The major reason for the visit was evaluation and treatment for a condition that supports the need for a hospital bed.

My clinical findings support the need for a hospital bed because:
The patient has a medical condition which requires positioning of the body in ways not feasible with an ordinary bed
Medical condition: _
_in order to alleviate pain.
_The patient requires the head of the bed to be elevated more than 30 degrees most of the time due to heart failure, chronic pulmonary disease, or problems with aspiration
_The patient requires traction equipment, which can only be attached to a hospital bed.

_Variable height - The patient requires a bed height different than a fixed height bed to permit transfers to a chair, wheelchair, or standing position.

_Semi-electric - The patient requires frequent changes in body position and/or has an immediate need for a change in body position.
_Heavy-duty extra-wide - Patient needs bariatric bed. The patient's weight is more than 350 pounds but less than 600 pounds.

_Extra-heavy-duty bed - Patient needs bariatric bed. The patient's weight is more than 600 pounds.
Accessories:

Trapeze equipment - The patient needs this device to sit up because of a respiratory condition, to change body position for other medical reasons, or to get in or out of bed.
Heavy-duty trapeze equipment - The patient meets the criteria for a regular trapeze but weighs more than 250 pounds.
Bed cradle - The patient requires this item to prevent contact with the bed coverage.
Side rails - The patient's condition requires this item and they are an integral part of, or an accessory to, a covered hospital bed.

,.f2f-oxygen

Face to Face Encounter Documentation

I certify that this patient is or has been under my care and that I had a face-to-face encounter that meets the physician face-to-face encounter requirements with this patient within the last 2 days prior to hospital discharge during this hospital stay. I have evaluated patient's oxygen needs.

My clinical findings support the need for oxygen at home because the patient has a severe lung disease causing hypoxia-related symptoms expected to improve with oxygen therapy.

Medical condition: _

Oxygen sat on room air of 88% at rest.
Date of test: 11/30/2018.
Test performed with a three step exertion testing (rest, on exertion, and recovery)

Patient is in a Chronic Stable state, exacerbations have been resolved. Other therapies such as nebulizers have been tried and deemed ineffective to maintain O2 sats, therefore patient will need oxygen to treat medical condition.

„.f2f-walker

Face to Face Encounter Documentation

I certify that this patient is or has been under my care and that I had a face-to-face encounter that meets the physician face-to-face encounter requirements with this patient within the last six months. The major reason for the visit was a mobility examination.

My clinical findings support the need for a walker because:
The patient has a mobility limitation that significantly impairs his/her ability to participate in one or more mobility-related activities of daily living (MRADL).
Medical condition: _

Beneficiary needs walker to perform MRADL's and the functional mobility deficit cannot be sufficiently resolved by use of a cane or crutches. The patient has demonstrated the ability to use the walker safely.

The beneficiary is able to use the walker safely and the functional mobility deficit can be sufficiently resolved with the use of a walker

The use of a walker will resolve their MRADL's.

_Patient needs a bariatric walker - The patient weighs more than 350 pounds.

_Patient needs a heavy-duty walker - The patient weighs more than 300 pounds.

„.f2f-wheelchair

Face to Face Encounter Documentation

I certify that this patient is or has been under my care and that I had a face-to-face encounter that meets the physician face-to-face encounter requirements with this patient within the last six months. The major reason for the visit was a mobility examination.

My clinical findings support the need for a manual wheelchair because:
The patient has a mobility limitation that significantly impairs his/her ability to participate in one or more mobility-related activities of daily living (MRADL).
Medical condition: _

The patient's mobility limitation cannot be sufficiently resolved by the use of a cane or a walker.
The patient's home provides adequate access between rooms, maneuvering space, and surfaces for the use of the manual wheelchair.
Use of the manual wheelchair will significantly improve the patient's ability to participate in MRADLs.
The patient has not expressed an unwillingness to use the manual wheelchair.
The patient has sufficient upper extremity function and other physical and mental capabilities needed to safely propel the manual wheelchair.
The patient has a caregiver who is available, willing and able to provide assistance with the wheelchair.

_Patient needs a Lightweight wheelchair - The patient cannot self-propel a standard wheel- chair in the home, but can and does propel in a lightweight wheelchair.

_Patient needs a Heavy-duty wheelchair - The patient weighs more than 250 pounds or the patient has severe spasticity.

_Patient needs an Extra-heavy-duty wheelchair - The patient weighs more than 300 pounds.

Accessories:

Elevating leg rests
_The beneficiary has a musculoskeletal condition or the presence of a cast or brace which prevents 90 degree flexion at the knee.
_The beneficiary has significant edema of the lower extremities that requires an elevating leg rest.
_The beneficiary meets the criteria for and has a reclining back on the wheelchair.

Manual fully reclining back
The patient has one or more of the following conditions documented in the medical record:
_At high risk for development of a pressure ulcer and is unable to perform a functional weight shift;
_Utilizes intermittent catheterization for bladder management and is unable to independently transfer from the wheelchair to the bed.

Anti-rollback device
_The patient self-propels and needs the device because of ramps.

Safety belt/pelvic strap
_The patient has weak upper body muscles, upper body instability or muscle spasticity which requires use of this item for proper positioning.

,.f2f-wheelchair-powered

Face to Face Encounter Documentation

I certify that this patient is or has been under my care and that I had a face-to-face encounter that meets the physician face-to-face encounter requirements with this patient within the last six months. The major reason for the visit was a mobility examination.

My clinical findings support the need for a Power Mobility Device (PMD) because:

Patient is being evaluated and treated for
_ morbid obesity and knee osteoarthritis.

The patient's
_limited mobility is causing lower extremity edema. Patient also has bilateral knee osteoarthritis causing pain with ambulation.

I certify that, based on my findings, the following DME is medically necessary: Power Mobility Device (PMD)

The patient's morbid obesity, knee osteoarthritis, lower extremity edema is limiting patient's activities of daily living by impairing functional mobility as in ambulating and transferring.

Patient's mobility is impaired in the home even though patient is currently using a walker.
Due to patient's _morbid obesity patient is not able to operate a manual wheelchair in the home. Therefore a manual wheelchair not meet patient's mobility needs in the home
Patient has the physical and mental abilities to operate a PMD safely in the home

_Pain in patient's knees and lower extremity edema limit ambulation.
Ambulation difficulty over time has progressed.
Diagnoses that relate to ambulatory problems: _Morbid obesity, lower extremity edema, knee osteoarthritis.
Patient can walk 10 feet without stopping.
Pace of ambulation is slow.
Ambulatory assistance is currently used: Walker.
Changes to require a PMD: _Patient is now developing superficial ulcers on her lower extremities due to worsening lower extremity edema and venous stasis dermatitis.
Patient's ability to stand up from a seated position without assistance is limited.
Home setting: _Lives at home with family.
Ability to perform ADLs at home: Impaired functional mobility as in ambulating and transferring.
Physical exam as above.

,.fail

Failed to change as expected.

,.insulin-sliding-scale-moderate

Correctional Insulin

151 - 200 = 1 unit
201 - 250 = 3 units
251 - 300 = 5 units
301 - 350 = 7 units
351 - 400 = 9 units
\> 400 = 11 units

,.insulin-sliding-scale-resistant

Correctional Insulin

151 - 200 = 2 units
201 - 250 = 4 units
251 - 300 = 7 units
301 - 350 = 10 units
351 - 400 = 12 units
\> 400 = 14 units

,.insulin-sliding-scale-sensitive

Correctional Insulin

151 - 200 = 1 unit
201 - 250 = 2 units
251 - 300 = 3 units
301 - 350 = 4 units
351 - 400 = 5 units
\> 400 = 6 units

,.medicare-pap/br*

G0101

,.medicare-prostate*

G0102

,.mirena-NDC

50419-423-01

,.nexplanon-NDC

0052-4330-01

,.nexus-letter-VA

To Whom It May Concern,

I am writing this VA Nexus letter at the request of my patient that has been under my care since _ for _PTSD and OSA. My patient's conditions are currently treated with medical therapy including _.

I have examined my patient's VA Claims File (cfile) and service medical records. I am familiar with his medical history and have also performed physical examinations over the course of his visits to my clinic, most recently on _.
It is my medical opinion that the veteran's _OSA is more likely that not related to his military service and associated with his service-connected _PTSD; the rationale being that my patient demonstrated no prior history of _PTSD/OSA prior to military service, as annotated on his medical entrance exam, and was while in military service diagnosed with _, and _test consistent with diagnosis, and was seen on multiple occasions for _. My patient reports recurring symptoms since leaving service and there is supporting medical evidence that _ there is an increased association between OSA and PTSD.

My patient's medical record demonstrates that the medical condition symptoms manifested in service and have been chronic ongoing medical conditions up to the present time.

Please do not hesitate to contact us if you have any additional questions or needs.

Sincerely,

,.paragard-NDC

51285-204-01

,.pet-companion-letter

I am intimately familiar with my patient history and with the functional limitations imposed by my patient's disability. The patient meets the definition of disability under the Americans with Disabilities Act, the Fair Housing Act, and the Rehabilitation Act of 1973.

Due to mental illness, my patient has certain limitations regarding social interaction, coping with depression, stress, and anxiety. In order to help alleviate these difficulties, and to enhance my patient's ability to live independently and to fully use and enjoy the dwelling unit you own and/or administer, I am prescribing an emotional support animal that will assist my patient in coping with my patient's disability.

I am familiar with the voluminous professional literature concerning therapeutic benefits of assistance animals for people with disabilities such as that experienced by my patient. Upon request, I will share citations to relevant studies, and would be happy to answer other questions you may have concerning my recommendation that my patient have an emotional support animal. Should you have additional questions, please do not hesitate to contact me.

,.procedure

Procedure

,.return

Return to clinic if symptoms fail to improve or worsen.

,.ros

All review systems reviewed and negative except for pertinent positives in history of present illness.

,.ros-full

Constitutional: no fever or night sweats.
Eyes: no changes in vision or eye pain.
ENMT: no ear discharge, nose bleed or bleeding gums.
CV: no chest pain or palpitations.
Respiratory: no SOB or cough.
GI: no vomiting or diarrhea.
GU: no difficulty in urination or blood in urine.
MSK: no muscle or joint pain.
Skin: no rashes or itching.
Neurologic: no headaches or tremors.

,.school-note

To Whom It May Concern,

Please excuse _Name from school on _Date.
Illness/Injury: _
Patient may return to school on _.
Please do not hesitate to contact me if you have any further questions.

,.signature

Dr. John Doe
Family Medicine
The Wonderful Clinic

,.survey-EN

Thank you so much for coming to your appointment and allowing us to participate in your health care. You will be receiving a survey soon. And we would really appreciate if you can take some time to give us some feedback about our service today. Our goal is to continue offering the best care and your review could greatly help us to continue doing so.

,.survey-SP

Muchas gracias por asistir a su cita y permitirnos participar en su atención médica. Pronto recibirá una encuesta. Le agradeceríamos mucho si puede tomarse el tiempo para darnos su opinión sobre el servicio que recibió hoy. Nuestro objetivo es continuar ofreciendo la mejor atención y sus comentarios podrían ayudarnos mucho a seguir haciéndolo.

,.time

Total encounter time was 40 minutes with more than 50 percent of the visit involved in counseling/coordination of care.

,.together

Shared decision-making was made with the patient.

,.triamcinolone-NDC

0003-0293-20

,.twimc

To Whom It May Concern,

,.uds-add

Addendum:
UDS consistent.

,.work-note

To Whom It May Concern,

Please excuse _Name from work on _Date.
Illness/Injury: _
Patient may return to work on _.
May return to work without limitations. / on light duty.
Please do not hesitate to contact me if you have any further questions.

SUBJECT INDEX

General Medicine
Advance care planning, 1
Chronic benzodiazepines, 1
Chronic pain, 2
CURES, 3
Diet counseling, 3
Fall elderly, 4
Fatigue, 4
Hospital f/u transitional, 4
Hospital f/u, 5
Marijuana, 5
Morbid-obesity, 6
Naloxone, 6
Obesity, 7
Opioids, 7
OSA screen, 7
Overweight, 8
Preop eval, 8
Stable, 9
Tobacco, 9
Transition of care, 9
Traveler advice, 9

Health Maintenance/Physicals
Health maintenance
 Female
  18+, 16
  25+, 17
  50+, 17
  60+, 18
  65+, 19

Male
 18+, 21
 25+, 21
 50+, 22
 60+, 22
 65+, 23
Physical Male, 24
Physical Female, 25
Wellness-exam, 26
Well woman check, 27

Physical Exam
Adult xshort-(no-touch), 29
Abdomen, 29
Cardiopulm, 30
ENT, 30
Breast, 31
Pelvic, 31
Rectal, 31
Testicular, 31

Cardiology
ASCVD score, 37
Aortic stenosis, 32
Atrial fibrillation, 32
Atypical chest pain, 35
Chest Pain, 34
Congestive Heart Failure, 33
Coronary Artery Disease, 33
Hyperlipidemia, 35
Hypertension,, 35

Lower extremity edema, 36
Orthostatic hypotension, 36
Peripheral artery disease, 36
Peripheral vascular disease, 37

Dermatology
Accutane, 38
Acne, 38
Actinic keratosis, 39
Alopecia female, 39
Alopecia male, 39
Alopecia areata, 41
Bed bug, 42
Cheilitis, 42
Claravis, 43
Cradle cap, 44
Cryotherapy, 44
Dermatofibroma, 46
Dry skin, 47
Eczema, 47
Folliculitis, 48
Folliculitis scalp, 49
Fragile-nails, 49
Granuloma annulare, 49
Herpes labialis, 50
Hyperhidrosis, 50
Impetigo, 51
Intralesional injection, 51
Keloid injection, 52
Keloid scar, 52
Lichen planus, 52
Melasma, 53
Mole, 53

Onychomycosis, 54
Paronychia, 54
Penile sebaceous hyperplasia, 55
Psoriasis, 55
Punch bx, 57
Rash, 57
Rosacea, 58
Scabies, 58
Seborrheic dermatitis, 59
Seborrheic keratosis, 63
Senile purpura, 59
Shave bx, 60
Shingles, 62
Skin tag, 63
Solar lentigo, 63
Tinea inguinale, 65
Tinea inguinale, 65
Tinea pedis, 65
Tinea versicolor, 66
Unna boot, 66
Vitiligo, 67
Wart, 68

Endocrinology
Acanthosis nigricans, 69
Diabetes mellitus, 69
Hyperthyroidism, 70
Hypothyroidism, 71
Low testosterone, 71
Osteoporosis, 71
Vitamin D deficiency, 72

ENT & Ophthalmology

Allergic rhinitis, 73
Cataracts, 73
Cerumen impaction, 74
Chalazion, 74
Conjunctivitis, 74
Ear lavage, 76
Epistaxis, 76
Eustachian tube dysfunction, 77
Glaucoma, 78
Hearing loss, 78
Mucocele, 79
Otitis, 81
Pterygium, 81
Sialadenitis, 83
Red eye, 84
Stye, 84
Subconjunctival hemorrhage, 85
Thrush, 86
Tinnitus, 86

Gastroenterology
Asplenia, 87
Celiac disease, 87
Constipation, 88
Crohn's disease, 88
GERD, 89
Irritable bowel syndrome, 89
Lactose intolerance, 90
Ulcerative colitis, 90

Hematology/Oncology
Anemia, 92

Lymphadenopathy, 93

Infectious Diseases
Cellulitis, 94
Dental clearance, 95
Hepatitis C, 96
Herpes genital, 96
HIV, 98
PrEP, 98
STD, 99
TB clear, 99
TB latent, 100
TB screen, 101

Neurology
Alzheimer, 102
Bell's palsy, 103
Cognitive impairment, 103
Concussion, 104
Cerebrovascular accident, 105
Dementia, 105
Dizziness, 106
Headache, 108
Hiccups, 109
Migraine, 110
Mild cognitive impairment, 109
Multiple sclerosis, 109
Occipital neuralgia, 111
OSA on CPAP, 112
Paraplegia, 112
Parkinson, 113
Quadriplegia, 113
Restless leg syndrome, 114

Seizures, 115
Spinal cord injury, 115
Syncope, 116
Tremor, 117

OB/GYN
Abnormal vaginal bleeding, 118
Bartholin cyst, 119
Colposcopy, 120
Contraception, 121
Depo, 121
Dysmenorrhea, 122
Endometrial biopsy, 122
Hot flashes, 123
Infertility, 123
IUD procedure, 124
Menopause, 126
Nexplanon proc, 127
Non-stress test/Amniotic fluid index, 128
PCOS, 129
Pelvic inflammatory disease, 129
Pelvic organ-prolapse, 129
Plan B, 130
Premenstrual syndrome, 130
Postpartum, 131
Pregnancy, 131
Prenatal, 132
Vaginal atrophy, 134
Vaginitis, 134

Musculoskeletal (ortho/sports/podiatry)

Acromioclavicular joint inj, 136
Achilles tendinitis, 136
Ankle pain, 137
Back pain, 138
Bicep tendinitis, 141
Buddy tape, 142
Callus, 143
Carpal tunnel, 144
Coccydynia, 145
Corn, 146
De Quervain tenosynovitis, 148
Dry needling proc, 149
Epicondylitis, 149
Fibromyalgia, 151
FOOSH injury, 151
Foot pain, 152
Ganglion cyst, 153
Gout, 154
Hallux valgus, 155
Hamstring sprain, 156
Hip pain, 157
Ingrown toenail, 157
Injection, 158
Injection knee, 159
Injection shoulder, 160
IT band syndrome, 160
Knee
 Aspiration, 160
 Injection, 162
 Meniscus, 163
 Osteoartritis, 163
 Patella tendonitis, 164

Patellofemoral pain syndrome, 164
PE, 160
Viscosupplementation, 163
Morton neuroma, 165
Mucous cyst, 147
Neck pain, 147
Olecranon bursitis, 166
Patellar bursitis, 167
Pes anserine bursitis inj, 167
Pes planus, 168
Piriformis syndrome, 168
Plantar fasciitis, 169
Rheumatoid arthritis, 171
RICE, 172
Rotator cuff, 172
Shoulder pain, 173
Splint finger, 174
Strapping
  Ankle, 174
  Knee, 175
Thumb CMC, 175
Temporomandibular joint syndrome, 176
Toenail debridement, 177
Toenail trimming, 179
Triamcinolone NDC, 179
Trigger finger, 179
Trigger point inj, 179
Trochanteric bursitis, 179
Ulnar tunnel syndrome, 182
Wrist pain, 183

Pediatrics

Circumcision, 184
Down syndrome, 186
Hand-foot-mouth disease-PE, 187
Obesity childhood, 187
Sports physical, 187
Well child check, Months
0-1, 189
01-2, 190
03-4, 191
05-6, 193
07-9, 194
10-12, 195
13-15, 196
16-23, 198
WCC PE infant, 199
WCC PE pub/teen, 200
WCC PE toddler/child, 201
Well child check, Years
02, 201
03, 203
04-5, 204
06-8, 206
09-12, 207
13-16, 209
17-18, 210
Weight and bilirubin check, 212

Psychology

ADHD, 214
Alcohol, 222
Anxiety, 217
Autism, 218
Binge eating, 218

Bipolar disorder, 218
Borderline personality, 218
Bulimia, 221
Buprenorphine, 221
Bulimia, 221
Depression, 221
Grief, 223
Insomnia, 223
Methadone, 224
Psychotherapy, 225
Suboxone, 225
Suicide contract, 225

Pulmonology
Asthma, 226
Asthma exacerbation, 227
Asthma exercise, 227
COPD, 227
COPD exacerbation, 228
Lung nodule incidental, 228
Lung nodule, lung cancer screen, 229
Pulmonary HTN, 229

Renal/Urology
Balanitis, 230
Benign prostatic hypertrophy, 231
Chronic kidney disease, 232
Erectile dysfunction, 232
Interstitial cystitis, 232
Nephrolithiasis, 233
Overactive bladder, 234
Phimosis, 235

Pearly penile papule, 235
Stress incontinence, 236
Vasectomy, 236

Surgery
Abscess, 239
Anoscopy, 241
Dental abscess, 242
Diastasis recti PE, 243
Excision, 243
Excisional bx, 244
Foreign body removal proc, 244
Global surgery period*, 245
Hemorrhoids, 245
hernia, 246
I&D abscess, 246
Laceration proc, 248
Lipoma, 248
Pilonidal abscess, 249
Post-op visit*, 250
Sebaceous-cyst, 250
Surgical tray*, 252
Suture removal, 253
Varicose veins, 253
Wound debridement proc, 241
Wound-debridement*, 253

Urgent Care
Abdominal pain, 264
Acute gastroenteritis, 264
Asthma exacerbation, 265
Bite, 265
Centor criteria, 266

COPD exacerbation, 266
Influenza, 266
Motor vehicle accident, 267
Pharyngitis, 267
Pneumonia, 267
Puncture-wound, 268
Puncture wound, 268
Subungual hematoma, 268
Upper respiratory infection, 269
Urinary tract infection, 272

Inpatient/SNF

Acute coronary syndrome, 274
Atrial fibrillation with RVR, 274
Alcohol withdrawal, 274
Asthma exacerbation, 275
Chest pain, 275
CHF exacerbation, 275
COPD exacerbation, 275
Cerebrovascular accident, 276
Death note, 276
Diabetic foot ulcer, 277
Diabetic ketoacidosis, 277
Diverticulitis, 277
Gastrointestinal bleeding, 278
Hyperglycemic hyperosmolar syndrome, 278
Hypertensive emergency, 278
Inpatient subjective, 278
NSTEMI, 279
Pancreatitis, 279
Physical exam adult ICU, 279

Physical exam adult, 280
Pneumonia, 280
Small bowel obstruction, 280
Sepsis reevaluation, 281
Sepsis, 281
Septic shock, 281
SNF chief complaint, 281
Soft tissue infection, 282
STEMI, 282
Syncope, 282

Messages: Lab, Imaging, Path Results

AAA screen, 291
Carotid US, 292
Colon cancer screen 292
CT lung cancer screen - nodules, 293
INR, 293
Lab results
Cholesterol, 294
Diabetes, 295
Hepatitis, 295
Measles, 295
Microalbuminuria, 296
Normal, 296
Prediabetes, 297
Testosterone, 297
Thyroid, 298
Vasectomy, 299
Lung cancer screen, 300
Mammogram, 300
Pap smear, 300
Pathology, 301

Path vasectomy, 301
Prostate PSA, 301
Strike letter, 302
UDS, 303
Urine culture, 303
Ultrasound, 303
Xray knee, 303
Xray normal, 303

Miscellaneous
Antibiotic delayed rx, 305
B12 injection, 305
Barbiturates, 305
Care plan oversight, home health, 306
Care plan oversight, hospice, 306
Diabetic shoes, 307
Disability paperwork, 307
Face-to-face
Cane, 307
Home health, 308
Hospital bed, 310
Oxygen, 311
Walker, 312

Wheelchair, 312
Wheelchair-powered, 314
Fail, 315
Insulin sliding-scale, 314
Medicare pap/breast*, 316
Medicare prostate*, 317
Mirena NDC, 317
Nexplanon NDC, 317
Nexus letter VA, 317
Paragard NDC, 318
Pet companion letter, 318
Procedure, 319
Return statement, 319
ROS, 319
School note, 319
Shared decision making, 320
Signature, 320
Survey, 320
Time statement, 320
triamcinolone-NDC, 321
To whom it may concern, 321
UDS statement, 321
Work note, 321

ABOUT THE AUTHOR

Dr. Bonilla was born and raised in Monterrey, Mexico. He received his medical degree in 2009 from the Universidad de Monterrey. After completing medical school, Dr. Bonilla served as director of Medical Education for a telemedicine company.

In 2012, he was selected as a UCLA International Medical Graduate scholar and completed his Family Medicine residency at UCLA-affiliated Northridge Hospital. After graduation, Dr. Bonilla was honored with the The Lillian Seitsive, M.D. Humanitarian Award for his outstanding humanitarian contributions within the residency program.

Dr. Bonilla is now a practicing family medicine physician in Woodland, California. He enjoys serving the Hispanic community of Yolo County. His practice philosophy is to empower his patients to take control of their health. He also strives to treat his patients as a whole, healing both body and mind.

Made in United States
North Haven, CT
05 June 2022